What To Do About Your Brain-Injured Child

Or Your Brain-damaged, Mentally Retarded, Mentally Deficient, Cerebral-palsied, Spastic, Flaccid, Rigid, Epileptic, Autistic, Athetoid, Hyperactive, Down's Child

OTHER WORKS IN THE
GENTLE REVOLUTION SERIES

How to Teach Your Baby to Read
How to Teach Your Baby Math
How to Give Your Baby Encyclopedic Knowledge
How to Multiply Your Baby's Intelligence
How to Teach Your Baby to Be Physically Superb

CHILDREN'S BOOKS

Enough, Inigo, Enough
Noses Is Not Toes
The Moose Book
The Wrong Cockatiel
Nanki Goes to Nova Scotia

What To Do About Your Brain-Injured Child

Or Your Brain-damaged, Mentally Retarded, Mentally Deficient, Cerebral-palsied, Spastic, Flaccid, Rigid, Epileptic, Autistic, Athetoid, Hyperactive, Down's Child

Glenn Doman

Avery Publishing Group

Garden City Park, New York

Printer: Paragon Press, Honesdale PA

Cataloging-in-Publication Data

Doman, Glenn J.
  What to do about your brain-injured child : or your
  brain-damaged, mentally retarded, mentally deficient,
  cerebral-palsied, emotionally disturbed, spastic, flaccid, rigid,
  epileptic, autistic, athetoid, hyperactive, down's child/ by Glenn
  Doman ; illustrations by David Melton.— [New ed.]
    p. cm.
  Includes index.
  ISBN 0-89529-593-8 (hard)
  ISBN 0-89529-598-9 (pbk.)

    1. Mentally handicapped children—Care. 2. Handicapped
  children—Care. I. Title.

HV891.D65 1994   362.1'083
                                                  QBI93-21547

Copyright © 1994 by Glenn Doman

Printed in the United States of America

10 9 8 7 6 5 4 3

CONTENTS

To my family, who believed me,

To the staff, who held the fort,

To those endlessly determined people, the parents,

and

To the brain-injured children—who live in

a threatening, frightening, and even dangerous world,

and who somehow manage to survive it all until help comes.

ACKNOWLEDGMENTS

There are four groups of people without whom there would have been no book and, for that matter, no Institutes for the Achievement of Human Potential. They have my love and respect which go far beyond the book; they make me the most fortunate of men. I list them with love.

> The Staff of The Institutes for the
> Achievement of Human Potential
> The Kids
> The Parents
> My Family

In regard to this particular book, I thank beyond measure Dr. Raymundo Veras and Dan and Margaret Melcher who made me tackle it again for the ninth time. For the illustrations, I am indebted to David Melton, father, artist, and author who made it easy by understanding it all. For the research, I am indebted to my assistant, Greta Erdtmann. For the preparation, I thank Vicki Thornber. The endless manuscript changes were made efficiently and cheerfully by Irma Kieslich, Cathy Ruhling and Sherry Russock. The original version was instigated and carried out by Lindley Boyer.

INTRODUCTION

This book of Glenn Doman is in many ways a very bad book. Upon my sober reflection, I see it to be the least good book of major importance I have ever read. However, perhaps this is so because I have not read many so-important books in my lifetime of reading. It is not so important to all people alive, but only of major importance to the parents of children.

This is not a bad book because to read it is difficult, for truth dictates that I report that it is very easy to read. Glenn Doman does not address himself to professionals but writes only for the parents, whom he so admires and respects. This makes it a marvelously easy book to read.

This is not a bad book because it is unexciting. His descriptions of the early discoveries of "the team," such as those which revealed the importance of the Floor to hurt children and normal infants, the reader will find exciting.

This book is not bad because it is not emotionally moving. The reader may find himself enraptured even to tears while reading the chapter *on motivation,* as I found myself moved.

I find this in many ways to be a bad book, because having started a New Age, he tells us so little about it in a doctrinal sense.

Glenn Doman gives us only the slightest glimpse into the years of unrelenting work through the brightness of days and the darkness of nights. It is a heroic story of a group of people who would in no case accept defeat and most especially when they *were* defeated.

This book tells us nothing of the years upon years of exploration into the lives of children all over the world. Glenn Doman does not tell of his expeditions and explorations into the wildest areas of the world, and they were many. He went so that he and his beloved "team" could see with their own eyes, while living with children, what no child expert had ever seen before since the beginning of time. He does not tell us how they have lived with children in more than fifty different countries, from the most highly sophisticated to the most wild. They have circled the globe at the Equator and lived with the great Masai in Africa and with the very small Bushmen in the Kalahari Desert in Africa. They have wandered over Africa, living with many tribes, and through the Middle East, the Holy Land and Asia. It was sometimes not very safe. It has almost always been uncomfortable. I know this because sometimes I have been privileged to be with them.

I remember a day, deep in the Xingu Territory of my own Brasil, where live the people who will one day come to the Stone Age, but who are not there yet by a long time. On this day, when the Brasilian Air Force had left us eight hundred miles from the nearest road and had flown away, we had marched for many hours toward a tribe called Kalapolo. The temperature was very high and there were clouds of biting mosquitos. I remember looking at Glenn Doman, Dr. Bob and Dr. Thomas. Their blood, from thousands of mosquito bites, joined with their perspiration to run down their bodies in rivulets, making of them a sight most fearful. They did not complain as they pushed through the tall jungle grass to see children and childbirth and child-rearing practices no child expert had ever seen before. Delacato and I being more dark complexioned suffered little from these nasty little creatures. But I have suffered elsewhere, having been with them to the Arctic to live with and study Eskimo children. The Arctic at 56 below zero F. is not the natural place for a Brasilian from Ceara. Of these storybook adventures, the book tells nothing.

Nor does this book tell us about the vicious attacks and terrible libels of fearful and jealous societies which the staff had to endure and fight off during the pioneering years. These unworthy enemies retarded for some years the work of the group, while they were developing the doctrines, the philosophy and the techniques which would give new lives to thousands of children and their families, not only in their own country, but here in Brasil and in other countries in South America, Europe, Africa and Asia. Although they have collected the fruits of victory, their continuing struggle for new knowledge and techniques give them no time to enjoy them. They have only tasted them. Of all this, the book tells us almost nothing.

This incomplete book tells us nothing of the world-wide search, in the beauty of their enthusiasm, for a single piece of the puzzle as to why it was that a certain group among the children, called athetoids, were failing to learn to walk even after years of treatment. It does not tell us of the brilliant deductions that led to the discovery of brachiation [using gravity to straighten rather than bend the body by using arms to swing from rung to rung on an overhead ladder] as a solution to the problems of those children and many others. In fact, it does not tell us of brachiation itself as the most important advance in treatment in twenty-five years, which has added an entire new dimension to the world of brain-injured children.

For everything this book says, there are a hundred things of importance it does not say. For every story it tells, there are a thousand stories it does not tell.

It is these things which make me say that in many ways it is a very bad book.

Contrariwise, I am forced to say that if this book told all the marvelous stories of the "team" and the rich, glorious days of The Institutes, which are worth telling, it would be a grand library instead of a small book.

I can't say that Glenn Doman knows more about children than any man alive, because I don't know every man alive, but I can say that he has *done* more about children than any man alive. I can say as well that he knows more about children—little ones and big ones—hurt ones and average ones—civilized ones and primitive ones—poor ones and rich ones—and how to make hurt ones well and well ones weller than any man I have ever read about or heard about or met. I know of no other person or group of persons who knew about all those kinds of children except him and the people he has taught.

Yet, Glenn Doman believes that every mother in the world knows more about her child than he does. Not only does his mouth say it and his heart feel it, but his brain knows it and he believes it.

He believes some unusual things for a professional. He believes in parents. He believes in children. He believes parents are the answer to children's problems, while everybody else believes they are the problem. It is easy to understand why he makes unhappy all professional organizations which earn their money from brain-injured children. He believes in fixing the children. Worse, he believes that parents can fix the children better than professional people. He teaches parents how to fix their children, not because to do so makes it economically feasible—although it does—but instead because he is sure that parents get better results than does any professional, including himself. This book *does* say these things.

He exists within a philosophical base very different from what we have formed through the example of our predecessors.

Most of all, he believes in results, and this book is the first book in history, to my knowledge, which tells how to treat brain-injured children, why to treat brain-injured children and most precisely what happened to a group of brain-injured children when they were so treated.

It is not only appropriate but also typical that he should write the first book in history which gives results of treating brain-injured children by a particular method in a straightforward, easy-to-read way. No other book in history has done that. Moreover, no precise results have ever been given of *any* treatment of brain-injured children before, with one exception. In 1960 an article appeared in the *Journal of the A.M.A.* on the treatment of brain-injured children with precise results. The reader may not be surprised to learn that Glenn Doman and his staff wrote that article also.

When we sum up this book we find that this is a book about brain-injured children and their parents. It tells *why* brain-injured children should be treated. It tells *how* the human brain can be treated and it tells exactly what happens to brain-injured children when you do it.

It is true to say that it is the worst such book ever written. But we must remember it is also true to say that it is the best such book ever written. The reason for this is that it is the *only* such book to be written.

It is very good for children—I think—that when it was finally written it was written by the man who knows more about the subject than any other man.

I think perhaps, in the beginning, the people who make books will not like it so much. Perhaps as well the people who are paid to criticize books will not like it so well. And, as I said in the morning, when I began to make this introduction, in many ways it is a bad book.

But I believe that many parents will find within this not-so-perfect book the knowledge and the courage they need to make their severely brain-injured children well without any further help.

I believe that many thousands of parents of the brain-injured, brain-damaged, mentally retarded, mentally deficient, cerebral-palsied, emotionally disturbed, spastic, epileptic, autistic children will find their own child within the pages of this book and will also find inside it the confirmation of their own heart's belief that he must have his chance to be free and will find the road to get the help they need to give their child that chance.

I believe this book will be the first true hammer in striking down the horrible institutions in which the brain-injured children of the world have been cruelly and unjustly confined.

Raymundo Veras, M.D.
President
The World Organization for
Human Potential
Rio de Janeiro, Brazil

1.

BRAIN-INJURED CHILDREN TODAY

On one Monday in this coming month, as on one Monday of every month, ninety-nine people will arrive at The Institutes for the Achievement of Human Potential in Philadelphia.

Thirty-three of them will be children with nothing in common except that all of them are brain-injured.

The other sixty-six people will be thirty-three mothers and thirty-three fathers who have nothing in common except a refusal to believe that their hurt child cannot be helped.

If it is a typical group, four or five of the families will come from Pennsylvania, twenty-three or twenty-four of them will come from the four corners of the Americas, and four or five of them will come from Europe or Africa, Asia, Australia or the Middle East. In short, from anywhere on earth. The children will range in age from one year to sixteen years.

Some will be so paralyzed that they are barely able to breathe; some will be so mildly injured that they appear to the eye to be totally well.

Some of the kids will be paralyzed from head to toe. Some will be blind as a bat. Some will be deaf as a post. Some will suffer from recurring violent convulsions. Some will be unable to talk or even make sounds. Some will have all of these problems.

They will come with recorded I.Q.s of 90, 80, 70, 60, 50, 40, 30, 20, 10 or 0. Most of them will be said to have unmeasurable I.Q.s.

They will arrive having been diagnosed as brain-damaged, mentally retarded, mentally deficient, cerebral-palsied, spastic, emotionally disturbed, flaccid, epileptic, quadriplegic, autistic, psychotic, hemiplegic, rigid, etc., etc.

Almost every one of them, on the basis of lengthy and sophisticated examination, we will diagnose as brain-injured, meaning that the problems are not problems of weak arms or legs, or poor musculature, or malformed organs of speech, or defective eyes as much of the world has believed. Instead, we will conclude that his problems originated within the brain out of some accident which occurred before, during or after birth, and that either interfered with the brain's ability to take in information or with the brain's ability to respond to it.

Of course, if the problem originates in a condition that could be solved by surgery—such as hydrocephaly—we prescribe surgery. However, operable cases will ordinarily have been diagnosed and taken care of before the child reaches us.

During the first two days at The Institutes each child is evaluated in the presence of the parents and each step in that process is explained. His every ability is measured against an exacting scale and precisely recorded.

The next two days, the parents attend an intensive orientation covering The Institutes' concepts and explaining *why* each concept, method and technique is included in the program.

Finally, on Friday, the parents go to each department of The Institutes where the department head shows each individual family exactly what must be done for each child and exactly how it must be done. At week's end, when the family has asked every single question they have to ask and when the last question has been answered, they return home with the child to carry out (if necessary to the exclusion of all other things) the program they have been so carefully taught to do. Every sixty to ninety days they will return to The Institutes for one day. During this day the child is precisely measured again using the exact same standards as before. Then a new program is laid out, and the family returns home to carry out the program for another sixty to ninety days.

Some of the children will be on this rigorous program for a year. Some children will be on the program for five years. Some others will be on the program for longer. Some of the parents will run out of energy and give up. Most will not give up. Some will never give up, even if they lose.

The great majority of children will do better than their parents had dared hope on the basis of prior experience with the conventional methods. With others there will be disappointment.

Sometimes a severely hurt child will make greater gains, more quickly, than another child whose problems seemed much less serious.

Some of the children who were completely blind will end up reading—not with their fingers but with their eyes like everybody else. Some will remain blind.

Some of the children who were completely paralyzed will end up walking, running and jumping—not with braces or crutches but with their legs like everybody else. Some will fail to walk.

Some of the children who were unable to make sounds will end up talking—not with their fingers by pointing and pantomime but with their lips and mouths like everybody else.

Some who writhed endlessly or could not remain still will find an end to their writhings.

Some of the children who were paralyzed and speechless and blind and deaf will end up totally well and in the same school and grade as their normal peers. In short, normal.

Others will end up walking, talking and dancing and perhaps with I.Q.s in the genius area.

The results, therefore, will range from total success to total failure.

It is not surprising that children sometimes fail in a world where most professionals were taught in school that hurt brains are beyond mending. Instead, it is surprising that anyone gets well. To many it would seem miraculous.

And who is it who has accomplished such miracles, if miracles they be? It is the parents who have done so, and at home. Parents—those commonly ignored, sometimes despised, frequently patronized, almost never believed people—will have done at home all of the treatment which brought a child from despair to hope, from paralysis to walking, from blindness to reading, from an I.Q. of 70 to an I.Q. of 140, from dumbness to speech. Parents.

In some cases, a medical doctor will be closely involved in the home treatment; over a hundred M.D.s have come and watched the work at The Institutes—and then enrolled their own brain-injured child. However, close to three thousand other families, quite without medical training, have brought us their hurt child and then gone home to carry out the prescribed treatments.

How is it possible for parents to accomplish this with their children?

Perhaps to understand such a process, it is best to begin at the beginning, which was really back in the forties. That's where we begin in teaching parents about brain-injured children. If one really wants to understand about brain-injured children, perhaps there is no place else to begin.

1940 to 1950
DECADE OF DESPAIR

Temple Fay, M.D., Neurosurgeon   Robert Doman, M.D., Physiatrist
Glenn Doman   Mae Blackburn, Administration
Hazel Doman, R.N., Pediatric Nursing

2.

TEMPLE FAY

When I entered the gleaming halls of Temple University Hospital & Medical School in 1941 to take up my new post as assistant chief of the Physical Therapy Department, I was considered by all to be fortunate to receive such an important appointment at a leading medical school at such a young age.

To keep the truth in perspective, however, it should also be pointed out that there were only two full-time therapists, the chief and me.

It should also be pointed out that my salary was ninety-five dollars a month plus meals for a five-and-a-half-day week, which, in all fairness was not bad for a physical therapist in those days.

To put the truth into final perspective, I was an eager but not very good physical therapist. Although I had graduated high in my class and had a high theoretical knowledge, I had had little experience.

There was one area in which I had absolutely no knowledge, either practical or theoretical, and that was the field of brain-injured children. It took me several years to find out that almost nobody else did either. In 1941 there were very few people who even claimed to know anything about brain-injured children.

Fortunately for me and for my future there was a man at Temple who probably knew more about such children than any man alive. His name was Temple Fay, and although Dr. Fay was then only in his early forties he was both professor of neurology and professor of neurosurgery. He was one of the all-time Greats of Medicine. It was in his service at Temple University that I saw and was fascinated by my first brain-injured child.

In those days, few if any people referred to severely brain-injured children as *brain-injured*. Instead, they were called by names like *feeble-minded*. This was because, being severely brain-injured, a high percentage of them could neither walk nor talk. It was assumed that the fact that they couldn't talk constituted sufficient evidence to prove that they weren't smart enough to talk. Even today most professional people assume brain-injured children to be stupid or even idiots—they were taught nothing to the contrary when in school.

I shall not forget the first brain-injured child I met. Being fascinated by all that went on and being aware of my monumental ignorance, it was usual for me to spend my off hours in the evenings going everywhere in the hospital. Because I was young and pathetically eager, department chiefs and head nurses opened the doors of their departments to me. Now that I am firmly entrenched in that period of life known as middle age, I realize how irresistible it is to be confronted with a person who is at once young and eager to learn. How powerful is the alchemy and how mutually marvelous the opportunity when one who is young and eager to learn meets an older person who knows something worth learning.

On this particular day I was in the nursery, not where the newborns (who also fascinated me) were kept, but where the very small, very sick children were kept. The children were in little cribs, and except for them I was alone in the room. I had read some of their histories and was now seeing the children. Most of the babies in the room were asleep, and the room was quiet except for the labored breathing of the babies and the sounds made by my white crepe-soled shoes as I moved quietly from bed to bed.

I was therefore more than a little startled, and I jumped visibly, when a voice said, "Hello," in a room where I considered myself alone except for infants and small babies. While the voice wasn't an adult voice, it certainly wasn't a baby's. I glanced hurriedly around the room and was extremely uncomfortable when I could see nothing but very small cribs.

Just as I was persuading myself that I had imagined the voice altogether, the small voice spoke again. This time I happened to be looking at the precise corner from which the voice came, and, as a result, I started even more violently than the first time. "What's your name?" the voice asked.

By now I was totally confused and more than a little frightened as I took three or four reluctant steps toward the corner of the room from which the talking was coming. I would not, even then, have seen him if he hadn't spoken again as I stood directly over the tiny crib in which he was lying.

"My name's Billy," said Billy, as I looked down at him. If it had been difficult to believe my ears, it was now even more difficult to believe my eyes. No one in neurology or pediatrics had ever taught me that such children existed. Looking up at me from a tiny crib was an extremely strange but not unpleasant adolescent face set in a head as large as any adult's. What shook me to the core was the fact that, although I could see the very large head, the rest of this child's body—covered with a blanket—could not possibly have been more than *two feet* long. I had the horrible feeling that he had no body at all and that I was being talked to by a disembodied head which spoke pleasantly and intelligently.

Although today, many thousands of brain-injured children later, I can honestly say that I have never once since felt horror at contact with a brain-injured child and am, in point of fact, quite upset by people who do, I must admit that I strove mightily to contain the horror I felt then. I now realize that it was not the child I was seeing that so upset me, rather it was not understanding the child I was seeing.

If I was upset, Billy was not, and his next statement gave me time to gain my outward, if not my inner, composure. "I'm eleven years old," said Billy, in a voice that made me think he had often answered that question. I do not remember the conversation that followed, but I do remember that Billy remained entirely composed throughout the ten or so minutes which followed. I have always hoped that I sounded more sensible than I felt.

When finally I managed to escape that room, I paused outside the door to calm myself before seeking out the charge nurse. I tried hard to appear nonchalant when I said to her, "Oh, by the way, what's the matter with that big kid . . . er . . . ah . . . that is, that eleven-year-old kid, Billy?"

I shiver a little as I remember that question and realize how it revealed my total ignorance. The searching look she gave me as she answered made it clear that the question itself completely revealed my ignorance. "He's hydrocephalic," she said steadily. "One of Dr. Fay's patients." She made both of these statements as if either one by itself explained everything.

I wonder now how I got the courage, but without even stopping to look *hydrocephalic* up in the medical dictionary, I took myself directly to the elevator and to Fay's office and asked his secretary if I might see him. It was an impulsive and astonishing thing to do since his appointment list was crowded with famous people. Fay had been called in to examine no less a person than President Franklin D. Roosevelt himself.

While I had made rounds with Dr. Fay, I had never actually spoken to him, and so large was his retinue when we made rounds that I had sometimes made rounds with him without actually seeing him. Since he was at the head of the long column, and I at the very end, I was frequently around the corner from him and received whatever physical therapy orders he gave me at third or even fourth hand.

I shall never know for sure why he agreed to see me and saw me immediately, unless it was his insatiable curiosity, whetted by the unlikeliness of my request.

In addition to everything else, Fay was a formal man in the old-fashioned professor mold, and it was difficult not to stand at rigid attention before his desk as his piercing eyes looked into me and, for all I knew, right straight through me.

I didn't give him a chance to ask me why I had come, but blurted out the question which was driving me to distraction and which had driven me to stand before this awesome person.

"Sir, I have just seen Billy, the hydrocephalic. What the devil is the matter with him?"

"The matter with him," said Fay, not answering my question, "is that he is hydrocephalic. Why the devil were you seeing him?"

Not even the clear rebuke in Fay's question could put me off, and after a brief and not very clear explanation of how I spent my spare time, I asked the question again. What the devil was the matter with Billy?

While I was obviously in trouble for seeing Fay's patient without his consent, it was equally obvious that something in my answer had pleased him. I later learned that nothing was more irresistible to Temple Fay than a young mind that wanted answers and that would dare to come to the right place to get them.

The great man explained briefly that hydrocephalic children had huge heads and tiny bodies because the cerebrospinal fluid constantly being manufactured within the brain was unable to escape, as it does in well people, due to a clogged resorption mechanism, and that the consequent increased pressure forced the skull to expand in size and compress the underlying brain. He recommended several books for me to read, although he cautioned me that they weren't entirely accurate.

Having thanked him for his time, I headed for the door. I had already partially opened the door when he stopped me to ask if my training at Penn had included experience in the operating room. I told him that it had.

"Did your experience in the O.R. include brain surgery?" inquired Dr. Fay.

In some intuitive way I knew that this question was a highly important one which could mark a turning point in my life. Fay's question had not been asked in a casual way.

I turned to face him. "I have never seen a piece of brain surgery, sir."

"Don't be so defensive, son, very few people ever have," said Fay, very deliberately. "Would you like to see some neurosurgery?"

Although he watched me very closely, he would not have had to, since the answer was obviously written all over my face. "Go see the head O.R. nurse and tell her you have my permission to come once. If your O.R. behavior suits both her and me, perhaps you can come often." He turned his back and dismissed me.

I couldn't believe my luck. The Dean of Neurosurgeons, Fay himself, had not only answered my question but had invited me to join him in the operating room. I was sure it was the first time he had ever seen me as an individual human being. He had called me "son." Did that mean anything or was it simply a synonym for young?

Fay had daughters but no son. I was to find that it was a term he used very seldom.

Being in an operating room with Fay was sheer delight. Not that he permitted an instant of nonsense. He ran a tight ship and he dominated that operating room for every second his team was in it. He did not dominate the situation because of his very high ranking position; he dominated it because he was Fay.

Fay was a Teacher. He was a born Teacher, he was a trained Teacher, he was a Teacher by design, he was a Teacher by choice, he was a Teacher by instinct. Most of all Fay was a Teacher because he could no more help teaching than he could help breathing.

I don't mean that he was a teacher, I mean that he was a *Teacher* in the same way that Aristotle and Christ were Teachers.

In the sixteen years of hours, days, weeks and months that followed, when for weeks on end I virtually lived with Fay, I do not believe there was a period of longer than fifteen consecutive minutes that he was not teaching me.

In all the years that followed, I do not once remember discussing the weather with Fay, even in blizzards, unless the weather had something to do with the brain or with a patient. If that's hard to imagine, I can only say that Fay was a man hard to imagine and impossible to forget. He himself was dominated by his own voracious interest in almost everything that mattered. I would say that he had contempt for all things that did not matter, but that wouldn't be quite true. It is closer to the truth to say that he was completely unaware of what didn't matter, or perhaps that he had some way of totally tuning out what didn't matter.

I had been completely hypnotized that first day in the operating room watching Fay caress a human brain. Fay was a superb surgeon. A few years ago a now-famous neurosurgeon told me that he had served under two very famous neurosurgeons, one of whom was Fay. Although he had always been furious with Fay personally, he said that one of those two famous brain surgeons was a true artist in the operating room and the other a bull in a china shop, and that regardless of how he felt about Fay otherwise, it was Fay who was the artist.

Even so, it was not Fay's brilliant surgery or even his love of that marvelous organ, the human brain, which made him the delight he was in the operating room. What fascinated me was his eternal teaching. He taught every moment he operated, beginning with his preparation of the patient, which, in later years, he insisted on doing himself, and ending not before he had personally put the patient back into the patient's own bed. One could learn more practical neurology and neuroanatomy watching Fay in an operating room than from any book or lecture.

There before my very eyes was the "beautiful and wondrous" thing he so respected and loved. Here was no dead, gray, ugly thing in a jar but instead the live, throbbing coral-colored human brain. Even hurt ones were beautiful to Fay, and so they became to me. In those days, a quarter of a century ago, there were not a great number of people who had ever seen a live human brain, not even among graduate physicians.

A certain way to arouse Fay's quiet ire was to let him hear an "expert" discuss the human brain familiarly if he had never seen a live one. Fay would note caustically that getting an idea of what the human brain was like from looking at dead ones in jars or photographs of dead ones in jars was very akin to getting an idea of what human beings were like from looking at corpses in caskets.

We had the extraordinary opportunity to see live ones, for in those days it was not unusual for a single piece of neurosurgery to require eight hours.

Apparently my behavior in the O.R. passed muster, because after the first time I was invited back again as often as I liked. Not only did I spend every moment of my off hours watching and listening while Dr. Fay performed his brain surgery, but indeed, I began to use the slow periods in the physical therapy department for the same purpose. By and by, I began to use some of the not-so-slow time in the physical therapy department, and as a result it was not long before I was called on the carpet not only by the chief therapist but also by the physician who was responsible for the department.

What the devil was the matter with me, they wanted to know? Didn't I know I was a physical therapist and had work of my own to do? Watching brain surgery performed by the master himself was interesting and all that, but when you had seen a few operations you had seen them all; but what was most important was that I was shirking my work.

They were right and I promised to reform, at least in terms of my working hours, which I did. But I still haunted Fay's operating room in all my off hours, including full time during vacation.

Still, I had to ask myself what I was doing spending all that time in neurosurgical O.R. After all, I was a physical therapist and a pretty junior one at that. Aside from the fascination of watching an artist work with his hands, aside from listening to a true scientist discuss what he was doing, why indeed was I wasting such a major portion of my life on this subject? There did not appear to be even the most remote relationship between what Fay was doing in the operating room and what I was doing in the physical therapy department.

Why was I gathering such large amounts of knowledge I would never be able to use? I did not know. I knew only that I was compelled, absolutely compelled, to spend every single moment I could steal watching Fay and listening to him. I was hypnotized. I was fascinated. I was intrigued. I was bewitched. I was hopelessly lost in what I was watching. Every day I was learning, although I had not the foggiest notion that ultimately his specialty, neurosurgery, and my specialty, physical therapy, would interact to provide new hope for brain-injured children everywhere.

Although I had no way of knowing it at that time, what I was seeing was the answer to what was wrong in the world of the children who had been written off as being hopelessly retarded. It would be a heartbreaking number of years before we would appreciate the relationship between those "beautiful, throbbing, coral-colored brains" that Fay was showing me and the children the whole world was failing so miserably.

Although I had not the faintest notion that it was so, it was the beginning of the beginning. A team was forming which would some day profoundly alter the lives of brain-injured children the world over and the lives of their families as well. It was a team whose work would lead it deep into the world of brain-injured children and beyond that into the world of children we presently call well. It was the beginning of a journey that would consume the lives of many people, some of whom were not yet born.

There was, however, much to suffer before that team would become a working reality. For one thing, there was World War II.

The morning after Pearl Harbor, I enlisted as a private in the U. S. Army. For the next four years I went from the Medical Corps to the Infantry, from the United States to Africa and back to the United States for infantry Officer Candidate School at Ft. Benning. In the course of infantry combat through France I became an infantry rifle company commander. Through the bloody, icy Battle of the Bulge and the struggle through Luxembourg, Holland and across Germany and the assaults across the Moselle River and the mighty Rhine and into Czechoslovakia itself we fought, we maimed, we killed, and we were maimed, and we were killed until we stood victorious. We had wounded, killed or captured many thousands of young German soldiers. Of an original company of 187 men and 6 officers, I had three times been reduced to 18 men and no officers. In all the world there is no greater pacifist than a victorious combat infantry soldier at the end of a war—unless it is possibly a defeated combat infantry soldier. Except for uniforms they are astonishingly hard to tell apart. The brains I had destroyed sharpened my desire to return as quickly as possible to my practice of healing rather than destroying.

3.

I AM PLUNGED DEEP INTO THE HEART OF BRAIN INJURY—AND DESPAIR

Although I did not know it, when I was discharged from the army in 1945, plans were being made for me by others.

Since the company whose command I had inherited during the war had been one of the outstanding companies in General Patton's Third Army, I had received a large number of decorations and the press had made much of it.

Back home in Philadelphia, the members of the Physical Therapy Association had read of this, and although they did not remember me, they read that I had been a physical therapist.

As a reward for what they considered my wartime accomplishments they decided to give me a ready-made practice. All of them were overworked and so each of them decided to turn over to me some of his patients. It was extremely kind of that group who later became my close and dear friends. I had never even heard of anyone who had been given a busy practice as a gift. It was a great compliment.

My new practice was, in fact, unique. It consisted of thirty-one patients, every one of whom had had a stroke. I would guess that nobody else in history had ever had a practice consisting entirely of stroke cases.

I was once again involved with the human brain—for a stroke is a brain injury, although we didn't think of it in any such orderly way in those days.

The vast majority of strokes are a result either of a hemorrhage due to a broken blood vessel in the brain or of a blood clot that lodges in one of the blood vessels which supply blood to the brain. The location, the extent and the severity of the paralysis that follows a stroke is determined by the location, the extent, and degree of the brain injury itself.

My new patients mystified me mightily. As time went by I grew ever more successful at keeping my stroke cases alive longer and longer; it was clear that the more active I forced them to be, the more healthy they became. But rarely was I wise enough to get them walking independently, even more rarely could I get the speechless ones to talk, and never was I able to make the curled and spastic fist of the stroke case into a functional hand. It seemed a strange thing to fail so consistently.

I recalled over and over again the first patient I had ever seen. This was before the war and just after I had graduated from school. He kept coming back to my mind unbidden, and at the oddest times, until remembering him came to annoy me vastly because if there had been something to learn from him, I had failed to learn it.

He was pathetic in so many ways. In the first place, he was old. In the second place, he was completely uneducated and poor as a churchmouse. He had had a stroke in his left and dominant hemisphere and a bad one. Thus, he was severely paralyzed on his right side and totally without speech. In short, this poor old gentleman had absolutely nothing, which was precisely why he had me. I was fresh out of school and had not a single patient. He was very poor and couldn't afford someone better.

I remember that his house did not have electricity and I remember, as well, that his family was just like him, which is to say that they were also desperately poor, had no education to speak of and were extremely simple people.

Full of enthusiasm and burning to help, I began to treat him. I did what I had been taught to do. I had seen plenty of people who couldn't move an arm or leg. They were mostly people who had suffered broken arms and legs and who had just had the cast removed. I had, in school, seen a few stroke cases, and we had been taught to treat them in the same way. So I began vigorously and enthusiastically to heat, to massage and to move the joints in his paralyzed arm and leg.

His family watched me in what was, I became increasingly aware, puzzled silence. After a half hour during which his son, his two daughters and his wife had several whispered conversations, his elder daughter, prodded by the others, finally dared to ask a question.

"We don't understand what you are doing," she ventured.

"Well," I responded magnanimously, delighted that the strained silences and whispered conferences had come to an end, "just ask me, ask me anything you like. I'd be glad to explain to you."

I was simply bursting with inner confidence, based on hard-won knowledge of every muscle in the body as well as its origin, insertion, blood supply and innervation.

"The doctor said something had happened to Dad's brain right here," she said timidly, pointing to a spot about three inches above his left ear.

"That is absolutely right," I said with complete finality. "A blood clot lodged in your dad's brain at just that point and that's just exactly what a stroke is."

"Then why," she asked, "are you rubbing his arm and leg?"

There followed a brief but thunderous silence. What I said to that poor and ignorant family was in every way inevitable. I was right out of school and filled to the very brim with modern knowledge and erudition. Indeed I was brimming over.

When I think of it now, which I do often, I burn with embarrassment.

"Oh," I said, "I couldn't possibly explain that to you. You have to go to school for years to understand that." It wasn't as terrible that I said it as it was that I believed it.

Who in the world in my position would have dared wonder whether my learned professors could have been so wrong and this poor, uneducated family could have been so right?

What I said to them, I still believe was inevitable. But if only, riding home in my car I had *asked myself* exactly the same question that they had asked me, namely, *why* in fact I was rubbing his arm and leg, we would have saved more than *seven* years.

I sometimes wonder where our work would have been today if we had known the truth seven years sooner, and my mind boggles at the thought. I know that a severely brain-injured child coming to The Institutes today has a vastly improved chance over a similar child who came seven years ago. I have an extremely active imagination, but I cannot for the life of me imagine what our world of brain-injured children will be like seven years hence. All I'm sure of is that we will know even more than we know today and be able to do more for more children.

But, unhappily, I did not ask myself why I was rubbing his arm and leg. I just continued to do so. I did so three times a week for the next fifteen months at the end of which time he was fifteen months older—but not even a little bit better. There was no real reason why he should have been better. What I was doing to him had a great deal to do with his symptoms, but it had almost nothing to do with the cause of his problem which was in his brain.

Somebody said once that ignorance did not consist so much of not knowing anything as it consisted of knowing so many things that aren't true.

That family was a perfect example of the former, and I was a perfect example of the latter.

Since I did exactly the same thing for my thirty-one other stroke cases as I had done for the old man, none of them got well either.

Perhaps I am too hard on myself and on those days because one terribly important advance had been made. Prior to World War II stroke cases had been kept in bed since virtually everybody believed that it was physical exertion which had caused the stroke in the first place and that the slightest physical exertion would cause another one. Because the patients remained in bed they very quickly developed hypostatic pneumonia or urinary tract infections as a result of immobility and then they died—not of a subsequent stroke, as almost everyone took for granted, but of hypostatic pneumonia or urinary tract infection.

Back in 1940, one of my relatively young stroke cases had decided that he would rather get out of bed and take his chance on dying than staying in bed and living. He absolutely insisted that I try to walk him. His doctor agreed to accept the terrible risk of letting the patient get out of bed. We did so and he improved vastly. We soon satisfied ourselves that it was the immobility itself that was killing people. So it was that in late 1940 and in 1941 we had gotten a half dozen patients out of bed into chairs. Moreover we had "walked" them around supported by two people. The more activity we had imposed on them, the healthier they had become.

Now instead of dying quickly they lived for years and years. But since few if any actually learned to walk or talk this only meant that they had more years in which to be depressed, despondent, morose or even suicidal.

These were the years of my discontent. I was now seeing five patients a day. Since each patient required about three hours of my time, it made a long day.

I massaged their paralyzed arms and legs, I used infrared lamps or hot packs or diathermy on their arms and legs to speed up their circulation. I moved all their joints in arm and leg over and over again to *exercise them*, although I always noted with a vague feeling of uneasiness that after I finished vigorously exercising a patient it was I rather than the patient who was tired. And why not? It was in each case I who had done the work. Following this bed treatment I would get the patient up and *walk* him around the room. At least after this walking we were both puffing. Finally, I would spend a long time just talking to the patient cheerfully pointing out how much farther we *walked* each day, discussing the news of the day. This was very difficult if the patient had a speech problem and I had to make a single conversation seem to be a two-sided one. I noted with concern that this business of cheering the patient up seemed to be the most effective thing I was doing. The patients looked forward with apprehension to my treatment but with pleasure to my visit, which roused them temporarily from their depression.

I also noted with distress that it became ever more difficult to pull them out of despair as the hopelessness of their individual situations became clearer and clearer to them.

There was an additional reason why these brain-injured patients had come more and more strongly to rely on me. This was that almost everyone else, including the people who loved them most, believed (covertly or even overtly) that they were either insane or mentally deficient.

I, on the other hand, living as I did with thirty-one *different* patients, had a unique opportunity to observe them.

Strangely enough, the more I observed these brain-injured patients with their agonizing frustrations over not being able to walk or talk, the more my opinion ran contrary to everyone else's. I found myself less and less able to believe them to be either feeble-minded or insane. The more time I spent in intimate contact with them the more I became convinced that they were not only intelligent human beings but also extremely sensitive ones and this despite some apparently peculiar patterns of behavior. Indeed, I gradually became convinced that highly intelligent human beings were more likely to have strokes than less-intelligent ones and that they retained that intelligence after the stroke although they were frequently terribly frustrated by being unable to express it.

It was obvious to these patients that I was deeply sympathetic to their problem and that I, and sometimes I alone, knew them to be intelligent and sensitive. This increased their dependency upon me to dispel their gathering gloom. It also increased tremendously the emotional strain that I was experiencing in the losing battle to keep spirits high. My patients saw ever more clearly the hopelessness of their situation, and so did I.

As it became more and more difficult to dispel their despair I began to feel a despair of my own and to ask myself if I had really done them, or the world, or myself a favor when by getting them up I had increased their life expectancy but done nothing to decrease their frustration.

By now the practice of getting stroke cases out of bed was becoming reasonably widespread, so that now there were tens of thousands of people who had been brain-injured by strokes who were not going to die but who were not going to regain much function either.

My patients spent the better part of each day crying, and more and more, I spent the better part of each night wanting to cry, and on occasion I did so.

It was almost good news when a family called to say, "We wanted to tell you that Mother died this morning and to say how grateful we are to you. Your visits were the high points in her life. They were about the only high points in her life."

Then I would say, "Isn't that nice. I'm glad her problems are finally over."

Then they would say, "Yes, we wanted you to know."

They were real *Alice in Wonderland* conversations, with life become problem and death become solution.

I was extremely busy, very much in demand, with my practice of stroke cases growing larger every day. I was possibly the most successful therapist around. I was certainly the busiest young therapist in the county. I prospered.

It was the absolute low point of my entire life.

4.

A RESEARCH TEAM BEGINS
TO SHAPE UP, 1947 TO 1950

I had not set eyes on Temple Fay, since a few days before Pearl Harbor six years earlier. I had in truth avoided him and I had done so rather consciously. The time I had spent with Fay before the war had been extremely rewarding—but it had also been expensive. All the time I had spent in his operating room was time that I could not be seeing patients, and nobody paid me for learning neurophysiology.

I had always considered it in exactly the opposite way. I had always considered it a superb postgraduate education for which I had paid not a cent of tuition. I would have considered myself lucky if I had had to pay a huge tuition. I had been privileged and I knew it.

Still, after the war I had avoided seeing Fay because a huge change had taken place. I was no longer a blithe twenty-two-year-old given to spending his spare time hanging around neurosurgical operating suites. Quite to the contrary and, I might add, in many ways much to my own astonishment, I was now a responsible married man much devoted to spending every non-working moment hanging around my wife, Hazel, and my son, Bruce, age one and a half.

I had met Hazel first when she was a child only eight years old and when I was twelve and therefore practically in my teens. She was the pain-in-the-neck little sister of my closest friend, Ray Massingham, who was actually thirteen and therefore actually in his teens.

It was natural that she would therefore become practically my own pain-in-the-neck little sister, and so she remained when I had gone marching off to war.

At Christmas time of 1942 I returned home from the African theater a lean, hard-bitten, bronzed twenty-three-year-old sergeant who had been sent home to be made an infantry second lieutenant. Then, quite as in romantic novels, I met my pain-in-the-neck practically little sister who had suddenly become eighteen years old and who was now a student nurse at Abington Hospital. We were married just before I went back overseas and just before she graduated from nursing school. Bruce was born in the year following my postwar discharge.

As a happily married man I had purposely avoided seeing Fay since I did not wish again to be hypnotized by him and by his work.

In 1947 I was attending a medical convention where I had hoped to learn something useful about stroke patients—but in fact had learned nothing—and where it had occurred to me that I might just run into Fay and get myself hypnotized all over again. I was leaving and congratulating myself on not meeting Fay when I met Fay.

He had me instantly.

I knew the minute he looked at me and through me with those penetrating eyes that if he had plans for me, I was a gone goose. He had made quite a fuss about my war record of which he had heard and said that he was pleased to see me. When he asked me what I was doing I could not resist telling him about my problem with my unique practice in *strokes*. After all, I had not the slightest question that this rather frightening genius knew more about the brain than anyone alive.

He listened to me quite closely and carefully. Fay, despite his genius (or perhaps because of it) was ordinarily a very poor listener, but at any rate he heard me through.

He told me that he too was quite interested in stroke cases and that indeed he had some very good ideas about the treatment of such cases. He had now left Temple University Medical School inasmuch as his brilliant and pioneering work in Human Refrigeration had become far too controversial for him to be able to remain within the walls of any normal institution of what is solemnly called "higher education."

I cannot resist a very small aside. There is no modern hospital anywhere on earth which does not daily use human refrigeration in one form or another—usually in many forms—to save human lives, to ease pain, and in other ways to improve the human condition.

There is not the slightest question that Temple Fay is the father of human refrigeration and pioneered it despite the bitter opposition, scorn and ridicule that the "recognized experts" so often heap upon any advance which they see as undermining their expertise.

He walked without fear in the pathway that had been trod by virtually every medical pioneer before him.

Ignaz Phillip Semmelweis, for example, had been driven to insanity by the prejudiced hostility of his colleagues after he proposed that physicians should wash their hands in a solution of *chlorina liquida* before delivering babies in order to prevent puerperal fever. (In the clinics of that time the mortality rate ran from *10 to 50 or 75 per cent among obstetrical patients.*) Semmelweis died in 1865, unvindicated in the eyes of many.

Another young man would begin an experiment in the very year that Semmelweis died which would vindicate Semmelweis posthumously and revolutionize the science of surgery. Indeed, surgery could hardly have been called a science with the horrifying death toll it carried until Joseph Lister introduced antiseptic surgery. Lord Lister died in 1912 but even his right to be called "Your Lordship" did not save him from the ridicule of his fellow surgeons who condemned him for advocating sterile operating room conditions and opposing what they termed *laudable pus.*

Fay with his human refrigeration or "hypothermia" was as ridiculed and condemned by his medical colleagues as were Semmelweis, Lord Lister and a score of other medical greats both before and since their time.

I remember that Fay's first human refrigeration machine used to sit in an old barn at The Institutes covered with dirt and pigeon dung and there it remained until he died. Today it is in the Smithsonian Institution where it properly belongs in belated recognition of the acclaim to which he had always been entitled.

Someone has said, brilliantly and succinctly, that "The first condition for immortality—is death." It is indeed.

But this was 1947 and Fay was a long, long way from his death and here I was, spellbound by him as I had been years before.

He had left Temple University in 1943 and moved his office to a spot near his home in the beautiful north Philadelphia suburb called Chestnut Hill. Here in a beautiful old suburban home he had founded an institution called, The Neurophysical Rehabilitation Center. Even the name was typical of Fay. It would be another quarter of a century before any but the brightest of his colleagues would begin to understand what that name really meant.

Fay was already working with several physical therapists of prominence, among them Milwood Mathers, Irene Neider (my boss and chief from Temple Hospital days), Roy Evans, a friend and classmate, and that most regal and charming of physical therapists, Eleanor Borden, whom I had known from Temple University days and who would one day join our team to spend the rest of her splendid life with us.

At any rate, Fay invited me to visit him to see what he termed some "new and exciting developments." It was all that I could do to keep from following him then and there as the children had followed the Pied Piper.

Fay was blessed with rare genius of a type that occurs only about once each century in any given field, but he paid for the blessing with a curse most dreadful.

It was Fay's fate not alone to be *misunderstood*, as is the case with almost all geniuses, but worse than that to be *un-understood*. It took me many years to understand more than a fraction of what Fay was saying. The reason for this I now realize was quite simple. When Fay was making every effort to speak simply and basically (which happened sometimes) he would usually still be speaking over the heads of the rest of us. Fay at his lowest was quite simply higher than his colleagues at their highest. They were his colleagues but they were not his peers. In fact, he had no peers.

As controversial as Fay was all of his life, he virtually never made a speech or taught a class without a *Standing Room Only* situation occurring. I have many times seen Fay speak when large numbers of people could not even crowd into the room or auditorium where Fay lectured and who yet remained to listen to his voice without once laying eyes on him. The audience was invariably enthralled, and despite the most crowded and uncomfortable conditions there was almost always the deepest and most respectful silence when he spoke.

His eagerness afterward to learn how he had done was almost childlike.

"Did they appreciate it?" he would invariably ask on the way home. His eyes would sparkle with warmth and pleasure when I assured him that everyone had enjoyed it vastly and that he had held them spellbound (which was almost invariably the precise truth).

"That's very good because it's important that they understand," he would say.

I would then summon every ounce of my courage, take a deep breath and announce with all the firmness that I could muster, "Oh, they loved your speech, sir, but I don't think that they understood a word you said."

He never did really understand why almost no one understood what he was saying. It always seemed so clear to him.

I left Fay that day at the medical convention enthralled and frightened. I was genuinely frustrated over my own ineffectiveness in helping my stroke patients and I wanted desperately to know what answers he might have, but I knew I could no longer afford to spend my time hanging around his operating room, what with a wife and family to provide for. On my own, I doubt I would have followed through on Fay's invitation. I reckoned, however, without Woody.

Woody (Milwood Mathers) was an extremely successful physical therapist who had been working with Fay in Chestnut Hill. He had, however, been approached by the Woods Schools to accept a position as the chief of their new department. The offer they had made him was an extraordinary one which he considered far too good to turn down. There was, however, a problem. He felt honor bound to continue his work with Fay until he found someone to take his place who was suitable to Dr. Fay.

I had been elected.

Woody had called me to make the grand announcement. I wouldn't be working *for* Fay but rather *with* Fay. He would rent me office space in the beautiful Georgian building on Germantown Avenue in Chestnut Hill which he owned and which housed his office. He would then refer his patients needing rehabilitation to me. I would treat them and would have the privilege of joining him in the operating room and in daily consultation.

As sorely tempted as I was to learn from Fay, it was out of the question. I lived on the Main Line, which was a western suburb of Philadelphia, while Fay's office was fourteen miles away in Chestnut Hill, a northern suburb. It would require hours of driving time daily. I was very busy both in my office and in my home calls. I had bought a lovely home and drove a Cadillac. I was a confirmed young family man and well on the way to becoming a pillar of respectability in my community establishment. I suppose that those days were as close as ever I came or will ever come in my life to being part of any real establishment. I sometimes wonder idly what it would have been like to lead a quiet, respectable, don't-rock-the-boat, establishment kind of life.

But Woody persisted in calling me each week, and it was one of those embarrassing situations which is obvious to all parties. On the one hand I was obviously being complimented by both Woody and Fay himself, and I was truly flattered by their attention. Still I knew in some innate way that even listening to his proposition threatened that whole peaceful way of life into which I had grown and which (after the horrors, intense excitement, physical pain, incredible exhaustion and acute discomfort of infantry combat) seemed so desirable by contrast.

I knew that what would happen to me if I visited Fay would change the entire course of my life. Why should I wish to change a life which was completely successful already?

Someone has said that conscience is that small part of you that feels so bad when everything else feels so good.

I wish now that I could say that the reason Woody finally got to me on the phone was because of my conscience. In conscience, I must say it was not. I finally acquiesced to Woody's importuning because he embarrassed me into doing so. I had each time pleaded being busy on every date he proposed for a meeting. On the final phone call he simply said that I could meet with Fay on the first date available to me.

Fay was too great a man and Woody far too nice a person for me to put it off any longer.

Dr. Fay's office was huge and impressive. It opened off a tremendous center hall. Just as I had feared, he was prepared to charm me into insensibility and fascinate me into mental flaccidity, which he promptly did.

We would have the opportunity to spend many hours working together (I loved that thought, but where would I *get* the hours). He would rent me the office across the hall for a very small rent (I was at that time paying no rent at all since my office was in my home). The office was very conveniently located for all the patients (but fourteen miles away from me and my present patients). He was sure I could earn more than a hundred dollars a week seeing his patients, which was a lot of money for a physical therapist (I was at that time earning more than twice that much seeing *my* patients).

It was a ridiculous situation for me and whether I liked it or not I simply had to refuse it for the sake of my family and myself.

"It sounds wonderful, sir. How soon can we begin?" I heard myself saying.

I tried at first to work in my new office from nine to five and to see my own patients all night long. It was physically exhausting, but that wasn't the reason my own practice soon began to disappear. For a month I strenuously resisted all temptation to be fascinated by Fay after five o'clock. But after a month this resolution went to hell in a basket. More and more I phoned Hazel at five to tell her to cancel my first evening patient, then I phoned to cancel the first two patients, and it wasn't long before all of Dr. Fay's promises had come true.

I *was* spending hours each day in consultation with him (instead of seeing my own patients).

I *was* paying a small rent (as compared to none).

I *was* driving fourteen miles to my office (instead of walking across my own living room).

I *was* earning the hundred dollars a week he had promised (instead of more than twice as much).

I was scared and in certain ways much more frightened than I had ever been during the war. For now I was intellectually frightened. I had never been intellectually frightened before in my life; awed by great people perhaps, but not truly frightened. Petrified that Fay would ask me any one of innumerable neurological questions to which I did not know the answer. Frightened that he would expect me to have treatment answers I didn't have.

But for all of that, I was exhilarated. Excited beyond any excitement I had ever known because now I was intellectually excited for the first time in my life just as I was intellectually frightened for the first time in my life.

Fay led me mentally into fields which I scarcely knew existed, let alone anything about. For example, never had anything prepared me to believe that what had happened to early creatures millions upon millions of years earlier might have the slightest thing to do with how human beings behave. All of my professors, all doctors I had met until now, all of my own professional people were extremely pragmatic and so also was I inclined to be.

If someone had a painful shoulder and you applied *diathermy* to his shoulder, and if afterward he felt better, then that was a good enough reason to apply diathermy the next time a patient appeared with a pain in his shoulder. As to *why* putting diathermy on a sore shoulder might make it feel better and thus "cure" it, the simplest of explanations would suffice. It was because diathermy "heated" the internal tissues and everyone knew that "*heat*" was good for you because it speeded up circulation and things like that. It had always been a good enough explanation for "practical" people like me and my fellow therapists and all of the physician fathers who had taught us.

Nobody had taught us to ask questions such as, "Is 'heat' *good* for painful tissues or would our patients have gotten well anyway? Would they have gotten well *quicker* without that heat? *Did* diathermy, in fact, heat internal tissues at all? Would *cold* possibly be good for painful tissues? Would it possibly be even *better* than heat if in truth heat *was* good at all?" Most important of all, nobody seriously asked the question *"Why?"*

Fay on the other hand was a master at asking "Why?" and this alone fascinated me. He made me think every instant I was with him, and nobody I had ever met before had made me think to anything like the degree that he made me think. Not only did he, in the end, force me to ask the question "Why?" of everything that I had ever been told and continued to be told, but he taught me that I had a whole endless world in which I might look for answers and that the only limit placed on me as to where those answers might be was the limit of my own knowledge—and he made me realize how very, very, very limited that knowledge was.

He made me realize that the answer to why my *stroke* patients rarely *walked,* almost never *talked* in a functional way and absolutely *never* used their involved thumbs correctly might not exist in the muscles of the leg, the muscles of the tongue or the muscles of the thumb. He taught me that the answer to those mysteries were not even to be found in the human being per se. He taught me to believe that those mysteries might be solved by our understanding of how the nervous system worked in a fifty-ton reptile—with a three-ounce brain—who had already been dead for millions of years and whose thunderous tread had not disturbed even the oldest of living things. But in order to look for answers to present human problems in creatures who had died long before the earliest human had existed, one had to know that such creatures had existed and had to know something about them. I alternated between wild hope at the new worlds his knowledge and genius opened to me and deep despair about all the things I didn't know.

I also alternated between getting to bed at midnight and not getting to bed at midnight, as Fay's demands on my time became greater. Even after going to bed, the discussions would often continue, as I poured out my heart and my exultations to my wife, Hazel—and received yet other viewpoints and ideas from her in return. Hazel had always been an immense help to me in the conduct of my own practice, and I found myself with constantly growing respect for the seemingly endless practical knowledge that she had acquired during her years as a student and graduate nurse. Of course, in addition to being confidante and colleague at 2 A.M., she was also appointments secretary and mother to our children, but before any feminist screams "Unfair" I cannot resist quoting Hazel herself. When asked about her attitudes toward Women's Lib she said, "I have always felt myself to be superior to males and I see no reason to accept equality at this late date."

Although I had now lost my own practice, I did feel that something important was abuilding to replace it, namely, a new and improbable kind of research team consisting of Fay, the world-renowned expert on neurosurgery; my wife, Hazel, who contributed two oft-ignored viewpoints, namely, those of nurse and mother; and myself, the physical therapist. We were shortly to enlarge the team by a fourth member, namely my brother, Dr. Robert Doman, who was just about to be released by the U. S. Army Medical Corps.

Dr. Fay had been feeling the need of recruiting a young physician he could mold early into his way of thinking regarding brain injury.

Fay himself was a neurologist and a neurosurgeon.

So it was not a young neurologist that Fay was looking for but rather some cross between a neurosurgeon and an orthopedist with a strong dash of physical therapist thrown in.

Precisely such a creature had just begun to emerge.

These new and strange creatures were called *physiatrists*. There were in the whole world only a handful of them. The few that existed were graduate M.D.s who had specialized in physical medicine and rehabilitation. Following their internship these physiatrists had to serve a residency as stringent and as long as a brain surgeon or any other specialist. Physical medicine and rehabilitation were themselves new terms in the 1940s.

The field of physical medicine was a gathering together of the three primary therapies used to restore function to non-functioning patients (rehabilitation). These therapies were physical therapy, speech therapy and occupational therapy. The physiatrist was trained in all these as well as in orthopedics, neurology and general medicine.

A physiatrist then would meet Fay's needs beautifully.

These physiatrists were being eagerly sought by every large hospital since, as a product of the war, new departments called "Rehabilitation" Departments were now a sign of a very modern and advanced hospital. Such departments were very rare, but most such departments were run by physical therapists because physiatrists were even more rare.

My brother, Bob, was such a physiatrist. We managed to get him before any of the many medical schools in Philadelphia could lay hands on him for three reasons:

1. He was eager to work with children, and Fay saw many children.
2. He was eager to learn from Fay himself.

3. He was my brother.

So by the end of the 1940s there were four permanent team members, Fay and three Domans, the last of them Robert J. Doman, M.D., Diplomate, American Board of Physical Medicine and Rehabilitation, and lately Captain U. S. Army Medical Corps.

Bob was a perfect addition to the team not only because he was a physiatrist but because of his temperament. He was the perfect choice to balance me. I have always been extremely fond of Bob and we have always had a typical "Jack Sprat" relationship with each other. While I am inclined to be quick to enthusiasm—quick to embrace ideas and inclined to solve problems by overwhelming them by immediate, direct and energetic action—Bob on the other hand is inclined to be more conservative, inclined toward an initial attitude of scientific suspicion toward new ideas and inclined to attack problems with deliberate regard. I have always been inclined to pull my brother along; he has always inclined toward preventing me from injuring myself in pratfalls.

Lest, in describing my brother's more studious characteristics, I make him sound stuffy, let me quickly point out that Bob is instantly beloved of all children—I have watched while Philadelphia children flocked to him, and have also seen him go down under a pile of parka-clad Eskimo kids in the Arctic, and several lapfuls of pre-stone age Indian children in the jungles of Brazil's Mato Grosso.

Children the world over take to Bob. He is himself, in the nicest way, childlike. I never saw a kid who got in the pool sooner than Bob or out later.

5.

A CATCH-AS-CATCH-CAN
ORGANIZATION

It was a loose organization if one could call it an organization at all.

Fay's Neurophysical Rehabilitation Center was avant-garde in the extreme. Too avant-garde. It was a patient success but an economic failure, and not even that genius, Fay, was able to act as medical director, chief, neurosurgeon, chief executive officer, director and administrator, all simultaneously.

In the end Fay's dream institute, born a quarter century too soon, died. The buildings were sold to become a nursing home, although some of Fay's patients remained and he agreed to continue to see them. So did I. Dr. Fay, Bob and I had our offices together in Fay's handsome Georgian building. I saw Dr. Fay's patients and Bob's as well. Our days began often in the operating room looking again at beautiful live, throbbing, coral-colored human brains. Our afternoons we spent together seeing patients in each other's offices or at the bedsides in various hospitals where we served as staff members. I often saw patients with Fay at the United States Naval Hospital in South Philadelphia or at the Hospital of The Women's Medical College or at Chestnut Hill Hospital where Fay now did most of his surgery. We saw clinic patients in many hospitals and we saw private patients in our offices, and I saw private patients in their homes as well. We saw children and we saw adults.

One thing our patients had in common was that they were all brain-injured (although we had not yet learned to call them that). Another thing they had in common was that, except for the acute surgical problems on which Dr. Fay operated, nobody ever got well. And this was no less discouraging because Fay had such fascinating theories about them.

We had actually founded what is today called a rehabilitation team, although in those days neither of those words was yet fashionable. Neither did we think of ourselves as anything so fancy as a rehabilitation team. I think really we thought of ourselves a good deal more simply and perhaps also a good deal more clearly. We saw ourselves as precisely what we were; a small but growing group of people each of whom was charged with responsibility for dealing with some phase of the problem of hurt children. Each of us was convinced he was failing the responsibility. It was for that very reason we had gotten together to form a sort of convoy to protect us from our mutual failures. Today that is generally called a rehabilitation team.

When we had begun our work together we had never seen or heard of a single severely brain-injured child who had ever gotten well. Nor did we meet anyone who claimed he had ever heard of such a child. Indeed, it is still possible to find professional people who become enraged at the mere suggestion that brain-injured children may be made to function.

If a man is going to choose a field in which to work, he cannot possibly pick a more promising field than one in which the success rate is zero and the failure rate is 100 per cent. Any slight change he can manage to bring about will of necessity be for the better. We had such a field.

Taken together we were seeing perhaps two hundred and fifty patients privately and more in clinics. All of the time we were learning, although as yet there did not appear to be the slightest pattern to this learning.

Perhaps the most valuable time of all was that which we spent together in the evenings after dinner, generally right in the kitchen of one of our houses. These sessions sometimes went on until it was daylight or until there was no more coffee or cigarettes. They were great sessions. They still are.

1950 to 1960
DECADE OF DISCOVERY

Martin Palmer, Ph.D.,	Speech Pathologist
Claude Cheek, B.S.,	Speech Therapist
Carl H. Delacato, Ed.D.,	Psychologist and Educator
Eleanor Borden, P.T.,	Physical Therapist
Charles Peterson, P.T.,	Physical Therapist
Lindley C. Boyer,	Author, Children's Books
Anthony R. Flores, Col. Inf.,	Physical Educationist
Thomas R. White, Maj. Gen.,	Legal Member, Board
Frank D. McCormick,	Director of Expeditions
Alice Letchworth, O.T.R.,	Director of Occupational Therapy
Jean Peters, R.P.T.,	Physical Therapist
Howard Peters, R.P.T.,	Physical Therapist
Florence Sharp, R.N.,	Pediatric Nursing
Edward B. LeWinn, M.D.,	Internist
Sigmund LeWinn, M.D.,	Pediatrician
Greta Erdtmann,	Administration
Daniel Cianchetta,	Engineering
John Tini,	Therapist
José Carlos Lobo Veras,	Patient (Brasil)
Raymundo Veras, M.D.,	Physiatrist (Brasil)
Elizabeth Galbraith,	Athetoid Cerebral Palsy
Mr. and Mrs. A. Vinton Clarke,	New Friends
Hugh Clarke,	Industrial Member, Board of Directors
Betty Marsh,	Practical Nurse and Impractical Financier
Jay Cooke,	Commanding Officer 111th Inf.
George Leader,	Governor of Pennsylvania and Board Member
Chatham R. Wheat, III,	Board Member
Rosemary Boyle, R.N.,	Charge Nurse

6.

A JOURNEY THROUGH FAILURE

By 1950 we had come to a moment of truth. By that time we had been treating a group of one hundred brain-injured children for a number of years. The children themselves ranged in age from one to nineteen years. They represented the types of brain injury that we felt we understood, as well as many types that we were quite aware we did not understand.

Many different methods of treating the disabled children were used then. Generally, a technique enjoyed almost universal acceptance for a period, only to fade a little as a new technique and a new hope was introduced and gained ground. The fact that so many different techniques existed did not mean that any of them were successful; indeed, it meant quite the reverse. The multiplicity of techniques in use was not a reflection of the amount of information available, but rather a reflection of the intensity of the search for a *better* technique.

The methods then in use included such treatments as heat (infrared lamps, diathermy machines, etc.) and massage of the affected limbs; exercise; orthopedic surgery to transplant muscles or to change bone structure to achieve various mechanical results, and electrical stimulation to help maintain paralyzed muscles.

Most institutions which treated brain-injured children used some combination of, or all of, the methods described.

Our team members were also using all of the methods described with great intensity, great dedication and great energy; yet hope was beginning to die as the years went by and few results could be seen.

The team decided it was time to evaluate honestly the results of our work. We decided that nothing but the brain-injured child himself should remain sacred. We carefully evaluated the one hundred brain-injured children.

The results of this study proved how tragically inadequate were our methods. For one thing, it quickly became obvious that we had never graduated a single child as being whole. If one were conducting a school from which no one ever graduated, eventually the question would have to be asked, "Is this school achieving its purpose?" Quite obviously our school was not.

Our hundred children fell essentially into three categories: (1) those children who were *better* following two or three years of treatment, (2) those children who remained essentially *unchanged,* (3) those children who were actually *worse.*

First we looked hopefully at the best group, those children who had improved, to see *how much* they had improved. We found our reports full of such statements as, "Johnny can now raise his head better." "Mary is less spastic." "Billy's balance is better." It was rather obvious that if it had taken two or three years of treatment, two or three times a week, to raise his head "better," Johnny was going to be an old man by the time Johnny could walk, and such treatment was not effective. So the children who were better were not better in any way that mattered. Many of the children had not improved at all. And, worst of all, many of the children were actually *worse.* This latter group of children was large, and there was no question about it, they were actually worse.

With a heavy heart, the team reviewed the question of why all this was so and what to do next. Our egos bruised by the tragedy of these results, we began to search for consolation, any hope, any reason that would justify the years of hard work we had spent on such children. An obvious answer presented itself. If the results of our work were slight, think what shape the children would be in if we had not treated them at all. Obviously, they would be worse. Much worse. We had at least helped some of them maintain the status quo.

Sincerely believing that this was so, we looked for a way to confirm it. There was a way. Over the years we had seen and evaluated many children who did not return for treatment. Mostly they were children who were in some way underprivileged. Some were children whose parents could not afford even our modest charges. Others were children whose parents simply did not care enough to undertake treatment. Searching our records, we found the names of those children and went to the parents, asking permission to evaluate the children again without charge so we might determine whether these children who had remained without treatment had indeed become worse.

We came to an absolutely astonishing conclusion. The children who had been without treatment were almost overwhelmingly *better* than the children we had treated! Among the untreated group of children, the better children had made more improvement than the best children in our group and the worst were not as bad as our own children who had actually gotten worse. The evidence was overwhelming. Not only was our work ineffective, but the children who had been without treatment were better than our children whom we had treated so long and so hard.

We faced a potentially tragic decision. Obviously, we could not justify continuing to treat the children if treated children did not do as well as untreated children. We had two choices. We could either stop treating children altogether and admit that all of our collective knowledge and work was of no avail, or we could find better answers.

We were unwilling to stop treating children. This meant we would have to start again at the beginning, on the assumption that we knew nothing. Indeed, was that not true?

Now each member of the team in turn was called upon to defend his methods and his reasons for using them. Each of the various specialists within the group had to stand still while the remainder of the group tore his field, his background, his techniques and indeed all of his beliefs to rather bloody shreds, for we had agreed initially that nothing from the past would be held sacred except the brain-injured child himself.

"What," the team asked the physical therapists, "do you do and why do you do it?" The physical therapist (namely, me) explained that he massaged arms and legs, that he gave corrective exercises to arms and legs, either in individual muscle groups or very holistically, that he did something called muscle re-education, and a team member asked, "Why do you do this to brain-injured children?" When the essential elements of his answer were finally bared, it could be said that he did these things for two reasons. First, because he had been taught to do so in school, and second, because physical therapists had always done those things. Perhaps, if one is doing what he has always done, because he has always done it, and is achieving splendid results, he can justify his work. But if he is doing what he has always done because he has always done it and the results are very bad indeed, in fact, worse than the results if nothing is done, he will have a hard time defending himself.

As each of the other team members in turn got up to defend his work, his defense was the same: He was doing what he did because he had been taught to do it and because he had always done it.

Again the team began long sessions of debate. The new series of discussions, however, had a new and somewhat frightening intensity

—an intensity that bordered on anger and indeed occasionally erupted into brief but furious quarrels. Only the mutual respect and admiration which the group had for each other prevented its dissolution. In short, the happy, enjoyable scientific discussions of good friends were ended and would not return until this specific question had been answered. For now we were milling about in the midst of a herd of sacred cows, and when a team member pushed a sacred cow aside, in order to get a clearer view of the world around the herd, he found he had best beware that the team's worshiper of that particular cow was not handled too brusquely.

It must, surely, be a difficult time for an African tribesman who has always worshiped the sun when he is being converted to a new and very different religion. Certainly there must come a time, a frightening and difficult time, when he is sure only that the sun is not the Deity but is not at all positive where or who the Deity is. Our team was in a very similar position. We knew with certainty the old ways didn't work, but we didn't know what would work.

We started again by looking at the methods of treatment we had been using and asking ourselves what they had in common. Certainly there seemed a very wide gap between massage, heat and exercise at one end of the spectrum and orthopedic surgery, bracing, crutches, casts, psychological treatment and so on at the other end. They had one thing in common, however. With them, every child in the group was being treated from his neck down, while every child in the group actually had his problem from the neck up. In short, we were treating everybody where his problem was not and nobody where his problem was.

We had to conclude that if one was to treat a brain-injured person, one would have to treat the injured brain, wherein lay the cause, rather than the body where the symptoms were reflected. Where did we go from here? Our decision was to begin at the beginning, throw out all existing knowledge and ask ourselves a very basic question: What were we trying to do? Obviously, the answer to this question was that we were trying *to reproduce normal*. Therefore, the only question remaining was: What was normal? To this question we now directed our efforts.

7.

WE SEEK HELP AND SO WE GROW

The question of what was normal proved to be a monumental one. In truth, it was a question we were not capable of tackling alone. There were many normals to be considered. All of us were predominantly expert in physical functions such as walking and hand use; we knew little of the fields of speech, psychology or education.

Help came first from a speech therapist: Dr. Martin Palmer, the founder and director of The Institutes for Logopedics at the University of Wichita. Palmer was an extraordinary man—physically huge, intellectually brilliant and in many ways as learned as Fay. He knew a very great deal about the human brain and this was what made him astonishing in a day when most speech therapists were orators who taught children how to project their voices. The few speech therapists who concerned themselves with medical problems believed that if a human being was speechless then he was either an idiot or had something wrong with his tongue.

Palmer and Fay were extraordinarily good friends considering that they were both unquestionably geniuses and that Fay was not a man who had many friends since he had virtually no social life. Although Palmer was not an M.D., Fay invited him into the operating room to share his knowledge of the brain. Fay, working from brain pathology which he saw in the operating room, could determine what speech symptoms a patient would have, while Palmer, working from a patient's speech symptoms, could tell what the patient's brain pathology would be. Although I was extremely unsure of myself, I was beginning, under the tutelage of both of them, to be able to do it both ways not only with speech problems but with other physical symptoms.

Martin Palmer flew in from Kansas at least once a month to join us in a brain-storming session. I was personally much impressed with Martin Palmer and his tremendous knowledge. He had a charming habit of saying something extremely scholarly, which was so erudite that I would have to strain to even follow the thought, and then he would look directly into my eyes and say, "Hmmmm?" Since the manner in which he said it left the clear impression that he was asking whether I shared his view (when in truth I barely understood it), I was deeply flattered.

We needed Martin Palmer full time if we were to answer our question as to what normal was. This was patently impossible, so Dr. Palmer did the next best thing. He sent to Philadelphia his most trusted student, a very young midwesterner named Claude Cheek. He was to supply invaluable information for several years as part of the team. Since his relationship to Martin Palmer was in many ways similar to my own with Fay, we had a great deal to teach each other. He was the fifth team member.

As for the psychological and educational aspects of the slowly growing team, these were supplied by Carl Delacato, who was to become my closest colleague for the next twenty years or more. So closely would our names become associated in the future that more than once in more than one nation on more than one lecture platform I would be introduced as Dr. Doman Delacato.

Carl Delacato had just gotten his Doctorate at my old school, the University of Pennsylvania, and was the headmaster of the middle school at a local private school. We had heard that he was a psychologist, that he was an educator and that he was extremely bright.

We issued him an invitation to visit us and he accepted. It was now 1952. Delacato was not yet quite thirty. Cheek was just past thirty and I was thirty-two.

Delacato brought yet another dimension to the team. Like my brother he was bright, mild and scholarly. Unlike either of us, he brought training and experience focused on the psychological and educational side of the normal child.

We could now find within the team wide and deep expertise of the physical, neurological, psychological and educational facets of normal and abnormal newborns, school children and adults.

Since we each knew our own fields reasonably well by now, we proved to be treasure houses of knowledge for each other. We made an exciting, stimulating and productive combination. For the next ten or fifteen years we fed each other's happy hunger. We did so in the brain-storming sessions over coffee; we did so on long walks. We taught each other in railroad stations and in airports, in classrooms, waiting rooms and operating rooms. We would in the future do so in South American jungles, African deserts, Arctic wastes and other unlikely places. We had a lot to talk about and there is no question that the new knowledge bred by this cross-fertilization was more than the sum of our individual knowledge. This was a case where one plus one did not equal two, but instead something a good deal more like ten.

A typical conversation went something like this:

GLENN: ". . . and so quite naturally the arm won't work."

CARL: "What did you say?"

GLENN: "Well, I don't know, I guess I said, 'So naturally the arm wouldn't work.' Why?"

CARL: "My God, is that true?"

GLENN: "Why, sure it's true. Everybody knows that."

CARL: "Like hell they do—psychologists don't know that! Why if that's true, we could . . ." etc., etc.

or

CARL: "So following Pavlov, the psychologists spent huge amounts of time carefully recording data about reflexes, time lag between stimulus and response and . . ."

GLENN: "The hell you say. Did they really?"

CARL: "Did who really what?"

GLENN: "The psychologists. Did they really record those data about reflexes?"

CARL: "Sure, tons of it, but everybody knows that."

GLENN: "My people don't! Good Lord, Carl, the therapists barely know that reflexes exist, never mind believing that reflexes have anything to do with their lives or their patients. But if the psychologists have already done this stuff and you can get your hands on it, we'll save *years* of work . . ." etc., etc.

And so it went for fifteen years or more until each of us had augmented his own expertise with that of every other member of the team.

Carl was the sixth team member.

The seventh team member was stately Eleanor Borden, already in her sixties and older than Fay, with the keenest humor and a true love for people. Eleanor was a physical therapist with the mind of a sixty-year-old and the courage and imagination of a twenty-year-old. She is today into her eighties and she still tells Delacato to stand up straight every time she sees him.

The team now grew ever-more rapidly as other physicians and therapists, fascinated by the work, came to see and stayed to work.

We were ready to tackle the first positive problem.

What, indeed, was normal?

8.

THE SEARCH FOR NORMALITY

In the beginning we sought particularly to understand the normal of walking and the normal of talking, since our children, generally speaking, could neither walk nor talk, or lacked at least one of these abilities. It was particularly the period from birth to twelve or eighteen months of age, when the normal child learns to walk and talk, that we wanted to study.

Our study began as most studies do, with a search through the medical literature to learn what had been recorded up to that time on the subject. We were astonished. Having braced ourselves for countless hours of studying the voluminous literature we expected to find, we were dumbfounded to discover that virtually nothing had been said on the subject! Gesell was all there was. It appeared that Gesell was perhaps the first man in all of recorded medicine to make his life's work the study of the normal child.

Certain it was that Gesell had studied the well child on a broad scale for that day, not only his movement and speech but also his social growth, etc. However, Gesell had not attempted essentially to *explain* the child's growth but instead had devoted himself to being a careful *observer* of the child and how he grew. But our group had a much narrower interest. Where Gesell recorded *when* the child learned to move and speak, we wanted to know *how* he did it, and *why* he did it. We wanted to isolate those factors *significant* to the child's growth. Clearly, we had to seek these answers on our own.

In an initial attempt to do this, the team went first to those people who might be expected to know. "How," we asked the experts, "does a child grow?" "What are the factors necessary to his growth?" We asked pediatricians, therapists, nurses, obstetricians and all the other specialists who were concerned with the growth of the well child. We were surprised and distressed by the lack of knowledge we encountered, but, on reflection, the reasons for this were fairly obvious. Rarely did the people consulted ever *see* a well child. Quite obviously the reason for taking a child to a doctor, nurse, or therapist is that the child is not well. Thus, the people consulted saw primarily sick children and rarely well ones. Consequently, we found in the literature and in our interviews with professionals that much information existed relative to an unwell child, but very little existed about the well child and why he grows as he does. We realized finally that mothers knew most about this subject. Even they were vague, however, as to the exact times that a child did what he did, and what was significant in what he did.

We decided to go to the source, the infants themselves. The world became our laboratory and new babies our most precious clinical material. We tackled walking first. If someone's cousin was having a baby, we went to that cousin and sought permission to look at the child carefully from the moment he was born until he learned to walk. What, we asked ourselves, were the things which, if they were removed from a child, or denied him, would prevent walking? What were the things which if given to the child in abundance, would speed his walking? We studied many, many new-born *well* children.

After several fascinating years of study, we knew we had rediscovered the pathway we had individually trod as babies. We also came to feel that we understood this pathway. In the dark and formerly unpromising tunnel we were beginning to see a little light.

Most particularly was it evident that this road of growth which the baby followed to become a human being in the full sense of the term was both a very ancient road and a very well-defined one. This road, it was interesting to note, permitted of no slightest variance. There were no detours, no crossroads, no intersections, nothing that changed along the way. It was an unvarying road, which every well child followed in the process of growing up. Anyone who could observe carefully could learn how a well baby learned to walk.

When all extraneous factors, all those things not vital to walking itself, were removed, the essential facts that remained were these. Along the road there were four terribly important stages. The first stage began at birth, when the baby was able to move his limbs and body but was not able to use these motions to move his body from place to place. This we called, "Movement Without Mobility." (See Figure 1.)

The second stage occurred later when the baby learned that by moving his arms and legs in a certain manner with his stomach pressed to the floor, he could move from Point A to Point B. This we called "Crawling." (See Figure 2.)

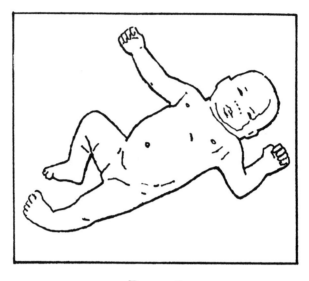

FIGURE 1

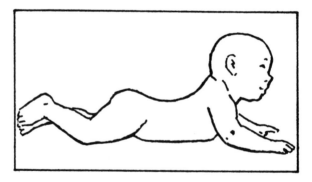

FIGURE 2

Sometime later, stage three occurred, when the baby learned to defy gravity for the first time and to get up on his hands and knees and move across the floor in this easier, but more skilled manner. This we called "Creeping." (See Figure 3.)

The last significant stage occurred when baby learned to get up on his hind legs and walk, and this, of course, we called "Walking." (See Figure 4.)

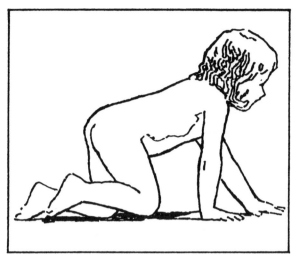

FIGURE 3

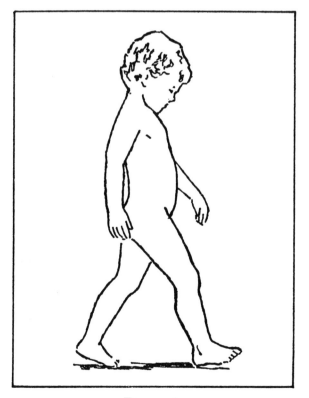

FIGURE 4

There is no hope of understanding the importance of what this book has to say unless the reader understands the full significance of these four things. If we viewed these four stages as schools, that is to say, if we looked at stage one—that of moving arms and legs and body without mobility—as kindergarten, if we looked at stage two—crawling—as grammar school, if we looked at stage three—creeping —as high school and then looked at stage four—that of walking—as college, we could see the importance of those factors. No child ever misses an entire school, no child goes to college before he completes high school.

There is an ancient saying that you have to creep before you can walk. We now felt safe in saying that you have to crawl on your belly before you can creep on hands and knees and that you have to learn how to move your arms and legs in the air before you can move them for crawling purposes.

We became firmly convinced that no well child ever missed a stage along this road, and we became convinced of this, despite the fact that mothers sometimes reported that their children did not creep. However, when such a mother was asked, "Mother, do you mean that this child simply lay in his crib or pushed himself on the floor until one day he jumped to his feet and then walked?" Mother generally reconsidered and allowed as how the child had crept for a short period of time. While there was no way to travel this road without passing each and every milepost, there was indeed a difference in time factors. Some children would spend ten months in the crawling stage and two months in the creeping stage while other children spent two months in the crawling stage and ten months in the creeping stage. However, always these four significant stages occurred in the same sequence.

Along the ancient road there were no detours for the well child. So convinced did the team become of this that we also became convinced of two other factors.

First, we became convinced that if an otherwise well child were to miss, for any reason, any stage along this road that child would not be normal and would not learn to walk until given the opportunity to complete the missed stage. We were persuaded, and we still are, that if one took a well child and suspended him by some sort of sling device in midair when he was born and fed him and cared for him until he was eighteen months of age and then placed that child on the floor and said, "*Walk,* because you're eighteen months of age and this is the age at which well children walk," that the child would, in fact, not walk, but would instead first move arms, legs, and body; second, crawl; third, creep; and fourth and last, walk—and that, therefore, this was not a mere chronology of events but instead was a planned road in which each step was necessary to the subsequent step.

Second, we became convinced that if any of these basic stages were merely slighted, rather than wholly skipped, as for example in the case of a child who had begun to walk before he had crept *enough,* there would be adverse consequences such as poor co-ordination, failure to become wholly right-handed or wholly left-handed, failure to develop normal hemispheric dominance in matters of speech, failure in reading and spelling, etc. Crawling and creeping, it began to appear, were essential stages in the programming of the brain, stages in which the two hemispheres of the brain learned how to work together.

To this day, we are convinced that when we have seen a child who did not go through each of the major stages in the order in which they are listed, however briefly they may have remained in a stage, we have seen a child who later on gave evidence of having a major or a minor neurological problem.

Now we had our first piece of certain knowledge. We knew what normal was, at least so far as mobility went. The next step would obviously be to determine how this piece of knowledge could be used to the benefit of the brain-injured child.

9.

THE FLOOR

We returned to our long-suffering, brain-injured children who had worked so hard and accomplished so little. Where, we asked, are these children along the pathway to normal? The observations that followed left us completely aghast.

We looked carefully at the facts and either did not believe what we saw or, perhaps, it must be admitted, did not want to recognize what we saw. The awful fact was that the brain-injured children *were not being given an opportunity* for normal development.

Gesell had described the floor as the athletic field of the well child.

The awful fact was that not one of our brain-injured children had ever been on the floor.

No matter from which angle we examined the facts, or how often, or how many excuses we made for ourselves, the fact remained that the brain-injured children had been denied the possibility to be normal.

We had come to realize clearly enough that a well child had to creep before he walked and crawl before he crept and would not learn to walk without the opportunity of working up to it by working his way through these stages. But we, the team charged with making the brain-injured child walk, were actually preventing his development by denying him the opportunity.

The brain-injured child, who had been treated intensively and extensively and with every device that anyone concerned could imagine, was rarely if ever given a single opportunity to be on the floor so that he might try to crawl and subsequently to creep and walk. It was an acutely embarrassing fact, but it was true.

If he was not on the floor with his well brothers and sisters, then where was our disabled kid? The truth is our problem child was almost everywhere except where he belonged. He was in braces, he was in casts, he was in a wheel chair, he was in a standing table, he was in a jackknife chair, he was in a special crib, he was on crutches or canes, he was in mother's arms; in short, he was every place except on the floor. Why was he where he was? *We* had put him there.

How could we have been so abysmally stupid?

Let's examine how we could have been so stupid. The arms of the goddess of tradition are enticing and seductive and so very comfortable. It is ever so easy to remain in her tranquilizing embrace and to do things the way she orders because it has ever been so. When one leaves her embrace to explore the region of new ideas, the climate may be brisk and invigorating, but it is also chilly and frightening.

Why had we built, for a child who couldn't move, an external skeleton of steel? It had all seemed so logical at the time. When we had seen a child who was four years old who could not walk, we had held that a child of four should be standing and walking, and if we could not make him walk, we could at least make him stand by giving him total or partial body bracing. This would be at least a step in the right direction. How sensible and seductive was this idea and how reassuring. Having supplied him with an external skeleton of steel called bracing, we could now say to ourselves with satisfaction (having stood him against the wall) that at least he was standing.

Looking at this child now, in the light of our present thoughts, we could ask ourselves whether it had really been true that he was standing, or was it nearer to the truth to say that he could simply no longer fall down? Could not a corpse be said to be standing under the same circumstances? By encasing him in steel braces from head to toe, we had painted an oil portrait of normality, but one devoid of life. It was a Pygmalion-like thing we had done. We had carved a statue of the child looking the way we wanted so desperately for him to be, and then we had tried to breathe life into it.

When we placed a disabled child in a special chair that resembled the letter "W," were we really placing him in a position that favored the improvement of his problem as we sincerely believed, or were we actually putting him in a sort of position of preferred paralysis which would make him easier to handle than he would be if he were in a totally rigid extension or if he were curled up in a ball-like position of complete flexion?

When we placed him in a specially constructed standing table, were we really strengthening his leg muscles and co-ordination as we hoped to do, or were we instead creating an illusion of normalcy which was pleasant to behold?

Even in those instances where the child was permitted to lie on the bed, crib or, rarely, the floor, he was seldom if ever permitted to lie in a face-down (or prone) position which might possibly let him crawl, but instead was placed, almost invariably, in the face-up (or supine) position so that we might be sure he was breathing properly and not smothering, and so that he might be amused by seeing the world around him.

How had it been possible for us all to fall into such traps?

It must be realized that until very recently there were no more than a handful of specialists alive who had gone beyond the mere treatment of symptoms and explored the origins of the many symptoms of brain injury. Consequently, very little information on how to diagnose such children existed. By the time the symptoms were recognized, the deformities which had resulted were generally very far advanced and the early workers in the field were, in most cases, orthopedic surgeons who quite naturally were thinking in terms of correcting present deformities and preventing future ones, rather than attacking the problem at its source, which was, after all, a neurological rather than an orthopedic one. As new workers joined the field, they had rather naturally learned from those people who had preceded them. For these rather natural reasons, the neurological disorder that had created the problem had received very little attention. A natural, but deceptive, evolution of treatment had resulted.

Having made an error it was necessary to correct it—to put the brain-injured child on the floor, stop all other treatment, and see what happened.

The results of this experiment were dramatic in the extreme and were destined to teach us many lessons we would never forget.

While many additional techniques and methods had yet to be developed, many of them complex and highly scientific in their conception and execution, none to this day has achieved nearly the significance of just putting the child on the floor.

When the children were placed on the floor, face down, we saw a reproduction of the exact stages we had seen in the normal child. The brain-injured children traveled down this road in exactly the normal order that has been described, without further treatment of any kind.

This explained, of course, the underprivileged brain-injured children who, it will be remembered, had done better than the kids we had treated so very hard with the classical treatment methods. Mother had not given us the opportunity to immobilize the child by treatment, but had instead taken the child home—placed it on the floor and permitted it to do as it pleased. It could now be seen that these "underprivileged" kids had pleased to crawl or creep. Underprivileged indeed! The children had instinctively demonstrated better sense than had our highly specialized world.

It was now 1952 and we had found our first method of treatment: *The brain-injured child who could not walk was to spend his entire day on the floor in the face-down position.* The only exception to this rule was that he might be removed from the floor to be fed, to be treated and to be loved.

Under this simple program we saw for the first time results we could really take hope from—tangible, significant, unmistakable results. Many of our brain-injured children improved more than they had in years. The results, however, varied, and in highly thought-provoking ways.

Some went rapidly from helplessness to crawling to creeping—but could not stand or walk. Some learned to crawl but not creep. And, of course, there were the children who had no purposeful movement at all, and could not take advantage of the new freedom.

In fact, although many children moved up a stage or two, they still tended to fall into one or other of the four categories we had noted earlier, namely:

1. Those who could not move their arms and legs.
2. Those who could move their arms and legs but who could not crawl.
3. Those who could crawl but could not creep.
4. Those who could creep but could not walk.

The children had stopped in the four precise places that we had earlier determined were essential to the development of normality.

However, they had *stopped,* rather than continuing on in the pattern of the normal child. The question was, what had stopped them?

10.

THE ROADBLOCK—INJURY

Now we were in the flood tide of ideas. Ideas flowed more freely and more quickly than they ever had before—so quickly that we could not investigate them all at once. Instead, we found it necessary to examine them one at a time, looking at each carefully while the others waited, containing our impatience to attack on all fronts at once.

The answer to the enigma of the brain-injured child was far from clear, but we had begun to erect the framework on which we could fasten pieces of information as we uncovered them. We now knew how kids who were well grew and developed and what happened to brain-injured kids when they were permitted equal opportunity by being placed on the floor.

We were particularly fascinated by one group of children. These were the children who had wriggled like a fish, crawled like a salamander, crept on all fours like a quadruped, but stopped short of walking.

Why could these children not walk? Certain it was that they crept freely. They could move arms and legs, they had balance, their bodies were good. Why did these children not walk? Certainly it would appear that these children had everything necessary to walk, and yet they did not. Why? Why? Why?

Suddenly, there the answer was before us, stark, clear and beautifully simple.

We had really learned the answer to this years before in an evening or perhaps in the distillate of a hundred evenings with Temple Fay. He was master of language and of storytelling, this brain surgeon, and he could shrink millions of years into an evening for us in explaining the function of the central nervous system. What he said to us went something like this:

"Every creature of the earth has enough spine and brain to perform the functions which he is expected to perform. He also has all of the nervous system possessed by all the creatures lower in the animal kingdom than he is. That is to say, he has what he needs as well as what all of the creatures which preceded him needed.

"If we take the earthworm, who is a simple creature, and therefore easy to explain, it will be seen that from a digestive standpoint he has a simple gut tube which extends from one end of him to the other. At one end he takes in food and at the other end he gets rid of waste products; he has a simple and effective digestive tract."

"Is his nervous system that simple?" asked a young physical therapist named Charles Peterson, who was now my first assistant.

"Perhaps simpler," replied the brain surgeon. "His nervous system is simply an arranged chain of neurons or nerve cells, which also run the length of his body. He puts out one segment of his body, anchors it down and then drags the rest of it up behind. Simple mobility; simple nervous system. It's all he has and it's all he needs because the earthworm is not expected to teach aphasics to talk, as you are," he said, nodding at Claude Cheek, "or to measure intelligence in a speechless child as you are," he said to Carl Delacato.

"Maybe my central nervous system is just an arranged chain of neurons, too," the psychologist grunted, "because I can't measure them either, and I'm trying."

"It is in a sense," the brain surgeon continued, "except millions of years more advanced and complex."

"Let's skip the millions of years in between and get to man himself," proposed Colonel Anthony Flores, a military physical educator who had become intrigued with our work. "What's with him? What's he do that's unique to man?"

"Well, of course, the end product of two billion years of evolution, at least up to now, is man himself, man who added the human cortex with the five functions we know it contains," said Dr. Fay. "It always shakes people up a little bit to come face to face with the fact that there are really only five functions that distinguish man from the animals. We may find someday there are others."

Someone ventured the thought that probably thinking was unique to man.

"Not thinking," said the psychologist. "We did experiments which are now ancient stuff with chimpanzees that not only think but even demonstrate deductive reasoning."

"But certainly one of the things that man does that the other creatures don't do is to stand erect," said someone else.

"Right," said Fay. "Standing upright is a function of the human

cortex. Man has a more fully developed cortex than any other creature, and he's the only creature who walks bolt upright in a way that
frees his hands for the use of tools or weapons. This kind of walking
is a unique function of the human cortex."

Bob, the physiatrist, added the next point, "There is at least one
function of man, and an important one, which I have to consider
every day. This is opposition: Man's ability to put his thumb and
forefinger together to pick up small objects. Man would be much
less man if he couldn't do this, and no other animal can do it,
although some of the apes come close."

"That makes the second function of man," said Fay. "Cortical opposition is a cortical function, and man is the only creature with that
skill."

"Don't forget man's most important function, that of speech,"
said Claude Cheek. "None of the other creatures come close to that
ability."

"I quite agree," said the brain surgeon, "although calling it the
most important is a somewhat parochial view and probably the psychologist and the others might feel that the other functions are
equally important. Nonetheless, speech is exclusive to man and is the
third function of the human cortex. The fourth is the other side of
the same coin, the ability to decode speech. Only human beings hear
in such a way as to understand human speech, and that also is a function of the unique human cortex.

"The last human function that we presently know is in your areas
of interest, Doctor," said Temple Fay, nodding to Delacato. "Know
what it is?"

"Sometimes I wish I didn't know what it is," said the psychologist,
"because it certainly causes me enough grief. It's the ability not only
to see the printed or written word, but also to interpret it in terms
of language. Only man can read language, and that too must be a
function of the uniquely human layers of the cortex."

"Yes, it is," said Fay. "So to recapitulate, there are five functions
that only man has, and they all exist in man's cortex. They are:

1. The ability to walk upright.
2. The ability to oppose thumb and forefinger.
3. The ability to speak and write.
4. The ability to understand speech.
5. The ability to read.

"All of these are functions of the cortex, and when you see a damaged cortex you will see the loss of one or all of these functions. This

is an important diagnostic tool never to be forgotten," said the brain surgeon.

Now, many years later, Fay's words returned. *All these are functions of the cortex, and when you see a damaged cortex you will see the loss of one or all these functions.*

Was this the answer to why our children stopped at different levels?

We rushed eagerly back to the children whom we had placed on the floor.

Were there children who had pretty much every function that animals have, that is to say all of the sub-cortical functions, but who stopped short of function at the cortical level?

There were some whose problem seemed to be focused primarily on walking; that is to say they could hear and they could speak but they could not walk upright even though their legs seemed strong enough. If their problem originated in damage to the cortex, it had to be damage affecting only the centers of the cortex controlling walking—so-called focal damage.

However, among those children who could crawl and creep but not walk, there was a larger group that could not talk, either. With growing excitement and enthusiasm we ticked off the things this group couldn't do.

Was this group able to stand upright?

No, they were not.

Was it further possible that this group of creepers-but-not-walkers couldn't pick up small items between their thumbs and forefingers?

No, either they could not, or they did it badly.

Had this group of children been able to talk, as well kids did, at one year of age?

No, they had not. When they talked later, they usually did it badly.

Were these children able to understand human language through their ears?

No, they did it badly or not at all.

Were these children able to read the language which was spoken by their families and which was their native tongue?

No, they read badly, if at all, even if long past reading age.

In this group of children, then, we had every reason to suspect damage to the cortex.

Interestingly enough, however, the histories revealed that even for such children as had in common the five symptoms spelling damage to the cortex, their backgrounds were very varied. Some of the children had sustained their brain injury before birth; some of the children had sustained their brain injury immediately after birth; others had been hurt by falls or disease at one, two or three years of age. Very different backgrounds, but all were damaged in the cortex or highest level of the brain.

We now had our first piece of vital information about injury itself. If a child, when given normal opportunities, got to the point where he could move his arms and legs, crawl and creep, but not walk, there was a great likelihood that his injury was in the cortex of the brain.

Now the logical question that presented itself to the team was this. If the cortex represented walking, were there other stages of the brain that represented the other three functions? Did the brain exist in stages, each stage of which had a separate, consecutive responsibility? After a long period of study, we concluded that this was exactly the case.

There were four essential and important stages of brain. The first, and the lowest of these, was that stage immediately above the spinal cord itself, called the *medulla*. This medulla was responsible for the ability to move trunk, arms and legs. Fish haven't much brain beyond the medulla, in a functional sense.

Next in order, and higher up, was the *pons*. The pons was responsible for controlling trunk and limb motion to move the body in crawling motions with the belly on the floor. Therefore, the pons was responsible for crawling. Salamanders and other amphibians, such as frogs, have a well-developed pons in addition to a medulla.

Above this pons was the *midbrain* and the midbrain had the responsibility of getting the child up on hands and knees in the first anti-gravity position. Therefore, the midbrain was responsible for creeping. Reptiles, such as lizards and alligators, have a well-developed midbrain, in addition to a pons and medulla. So do higher quadrupeds.

Finally, as has been said, the cortex, or top of the brain, was responsible, among other things, for the human ability to walk.

The team came to these conclusions after a lengthy search of the records. We started with the records of our own children and went from there to hospitals where we spent weeks poking into the records rooms (which were seldom the most attractive areas of such institutions and in those days were generally located in dusty and crowded basements). We sat on the floor of crowded records rooms going over dusty records with the absorption of a Sherlock Holmes uncovering obscure clues. The comparison to a piece of detective work is perhaps an apt one, for a search of medical records can tell a terribly interesting story to people attuned to what may be in them. Although long periods of sitting on a cold floor may result in what we described as double-feature paralysis, it was a small price to pay for the results.

In almost every case where records of test results could be found, they confirmed our belief. Wherever we were able to verify the existence of damage to the cortex (usually through surgery or autopsy), we found a record of loss of one or all the distinctively cortical functions enumerated by Fay.

Again the team knew the satisfaction of a hard-won victory. Again there was a period of elation and again a rededication to the job ahead with new energy born now of success. We had established another principle.

We called this new method of determining the stage of brain injury by a somewhat fancy but nonetheless descriptive title: *Functional Neurological Diagnosis*. Through the years we would continue to add to, to refine and to sophisticate the symptoms of varying levels of brain injury, but none of the dozens of future additions, refinements or sophistication would bring us nearly the excitement or satisfaction that we found in the basic discovery that we could diagnose a brain-injured child's level of brain injury by examining what he could not do.

11.

PATTERNING

Now, in addition to knowing that if a child were injured at any of the stages described he would stop progressing at that stage, we also knew that he could not progress beyond that stage even though he was not damaged at higher stages. Therefore, if the child were hurt at midbrain he would not only be unable to creep, but because he was not able to creep he would also not be able to walk, since creeping is necessary before walking can take place, as we had proved in our study of well children.

The team was now faced with *the* question: Must we accept defeat? If a child were hurt in the midbrain, did it mean that this child could never creep and therefore never walk, or was there something we could do about this? Was it possible, we asked ourselves, to build a bridge, if you like, across this injury? Could we dig a tunnel or beat our way through the injured midbrain? Could we, perhaps, go back to the point at which Nature had accepted defeat and simply intensify those sensory inputs which had clearly fallen short of doing their job but might not have fallen *far* short?

We knew the lower stages of the pons, the medulla and cord to be intact because we could check the movements they control. Now, was there a way we could check his higher stages beyond midbrain when we had made the decision that it was true that his midbrain was hurt? If his midbrain was hurt, he would not walk; therefore did that mean that we could not check to see if his cortex was intact?

Well, we knew that there were five functions of the cortex, only one of which was walking. Therefore, if we checked the other four in a child who could not walk or creep because he was hurt in the midbrain, would we find that he could nonetheless perform the other four cortical functions? Suppose that he could speak, suppose that he could read, suppose that he could oppose his thumb and forefinger and suppose that he could understand human speech. Did it not seem extremely likely that this child was good in the cortex since four of his five cortical functions were intact? Might it not also be assumed that the fifth, that of walking, was wanting only because he was unable to creep? This did appear to be a logical assumption, and we knew that the only time there might be an exception to this would be if a child had, in addition to the midbrain injury, a highly localized injury confined purely to that area of his cortex that is responsible for walking itself.

Could we now do something about this hurt midbrain? (Of course we knew that we never saw a child who was *minus* a midbrain; a child could not live without one. We were seeing only children who had *hurt* midbrains and, obviously, this degree of hurt varied from a little bit of hurt to a great deal.)

Suppose, we finally asked ourselves, we tried to teach his hurt midbrain the functions that it would have performed had it *not* been hurt?

In the past, we had tried to teach muscles, but the very term *muscle re-education* was a contradiction in terms, in that it implied that a muscle had the capacity to learn. A muscle is simply a piece of meat and is in every sense uneducable. On the other hand, if we tried to teach the hurt stage of *brain* its *own* function rather than to attempt to teach the *muscle* an *exercise* . . . was this a possibility? Could we teach the hurt midbrain its function of creeping?

Again we returned to the well children to study carefully the things that the well child did, in order to determine what creeping looked like. Having watched the normal child creep on hands and knees, we carefully recorded the separate functions of each of his bodily parts in the symphonious whole. We could then proceed to try to superimpose this ability on the hurt brain which, because it was hurt, was unable to perform its own function.

Creeping differs from crawling in that it not only rewards co-ordination but requires it. A creature that drags along on its stomach can move its four legs more or less at random and still make progress. A creature that has lifted its body from the ground must learn, however, *not* to pick up both right legs or both front legs at the same time —or it will fall. Efficiency requires picking up the right front leg only in combination with the left rear leg, or vice-versa, in a cross-pattern type of co-ordination. Only creatures with midbrains have this skill.

Temple Fay had long ago used the term *cross pattern* in his studies of how the lizard or alligator, both midbrain creatures, moved. He had even developed different ways of putting brain-injured children through the same motions, a procedure he called "patterning." This patterning had appeared to help but as applied had not actually succeeded in getting paralyzed children to walk. We decided to try again. We altered his patterns somewhat to represent how a well child moved, in contrast to how a reptile moved, although there were many similarities between the two. We stepped up the frequency of the patternings, remembering how much of his time a well baby spends in going through these motions. We then began the administration of those patterns.

Let me review our logic here. Fay had stated that each creature's brain embraces those capabilities it needs for survival plus those capabilities each creature lower on the evolutionary scale had needed for its survival. The lizard does not reason out the advantages of cross-pattern walking. He is simply endowed with a brain that lets him walk in cross pattern without having to think about it. We, as his descendants, still have that built-in instinct for cross-pattern locomotion. With our "patterning," all we were trying to do was to awaken those inherited instincts.

In a well child, the reflexes produce movement which he can feel. What he feels develops his capacity to feel, and matures the sensory portions of his brain. As the brain matures it begins to appreciate the correlation between motor output and sensory response. It becomes able to initiate voluntarily an action that was originally reflex. Each additional cycle matures both the intake and output portions of the brain.

In the case of a child who had failed, for any reason, to complete this cycle on his own, could we perhaps give him external help? Instead of relying wholly on the random reflexes to teach his brain how motion feels, could we perhaps impose the motions from without and thus give his brain an exposure to the feel of motion that would be even more purposeful and greatly intensified?

We decided to try it. In the case of a child with a midbrain injury, who could not move his arms and legs purposefully when on his belly, we decided to try moving those arms and legs for him—and in the exact pattern that the midbrain was designed for. We decided to "pattern" him.

The patterns were administered by three adults, and were to be performed smoothly and rhythmically. One adult turned the head, while the adult on the side toward which the head was turned flexed the arm and extended the leg. The adult on the opposite side extended the arm and flexed the leg. When the head was turned the other way, the position of the limbs was reversed. Through the years the basic pattern has remained the same, with only slight modifications. We found eventually that when this patterning was done often enough, consistently enough and in a time pattern, which we made more rigid as time went on, then indeed many a child with a hurt midbrain would begin to creep and, indeed, once creeping began, walking followed since it was normal to his well cortex.

We had now answered, at least for those people hurt in the midbrain, a terribly important question. Could we actually treat such people? The answer was yes.

If treatment implies actually changing illness itself, then indeed this was our first *true* treatment method, as opposed to merely giving normal opportunity, which we accomplished when we put the children on the floor, important as that might be.

Now it remained to be determined whether we could develop like procedures for the other brain areas, by imitating precisely the things a well child did as he went through each of these stages. With this question in mind, we now moved back down the scale to determine whether there was a method that we could use to superimpose the normal crawling methods on the brain of the pons-injured child.

Again we examined carefully the well child, this time as he went through the pons stage or crawling stage (usually at around five months of age). Again, after many attempts and many failures, we developed a method that was very similar to the method used by Fay, whose brilliant conclusions regarding the amphibians we now paralleled with the normal movements of well children. This pattern of activity he had long ago called *homolateral patterning,* and this appeared to us to be a good name.

This pattern was also administered by three adults. One adult turned the head, while the adult on the side to which the head was turned flexed the arm and leg. The adult on the opposite side extended both limbs. As the head was turned, the flexed limbs extended while the extended limbs flexed. We found that when this pattern was administered rigidly enough and frequently enough, in a timed pattern, many of the children hurt in the pons began to crawl. When they became able to crawl, if their midbrain and cortex were uninjured, they would rapidly move through creeping to walking and do well. (It is interesting to note that of all the methods of patterning that had been described by Temple Fay in his study of the growth of the race, the homolateral pattern is the only one which has remained almost exactly as he described it in his original work.)

Now there remained only the bottom and the top—the medulla and cord, and the cortex. We turned our attention first to the medulla and cord, the lowest stage of brain, which controlled the very basic first movements of arms and legs that precede crawling.

As has been said earlier, if a well infant, in the days immediately following birth, is placed on its face instead of on its back, one can observe the normal movement of arms and legs. Though these movements do not result in crawling at this stage of the game, they are synchronous movements of both trunk and limbs which *aim in the direction of crawling*. Here again we devised a pattern of movement. We called it *truncal movement*. Again the head was turned by one adult while an adult worked on each side of the body. When the head was turned to the left, the left shoulder and hip were lifted a few inches off the table. When the head was turned to the right, the right shoulder and hip were lifted and the left shoulder and hip were brought to rest on the table.

Again success was achieved in many children.

Now there remained only the question of whether or not we could reproduce the final stage of walking in children hurt in the cortex. It seemed strange to us, initially, that this was the most difficult of all the problems to solve, although as time went by the reasons became increasingly apparent.

We had studied walking in the well baby in intricate detail—in particular those things that had followed creeping but preceded normal walking. The well baby, in between creeping and totally well walking, did many things. Among these was getting onto his knees and walking for brief periods of time on his knees. He also pulled himself up by holding onto furniture and walked holding onto furniture. He also experimented by getting up in the middle of the floor all by himself in a position, not of hands and knees, but of hands and feet in a sort of inverted "U" and from there attempted to stand unsupported. This last stage Fay had described as *elephant walking,* and he had felt this was useful since it was a stage that occurred in man's phylogenetic growth. Although we tried this repeatedly as a technique to precede walking, we did not get useful results even though we saw well children do this frequently. We did find, however, that walking on the knees could sometimes be a helpful prelude to walking itself, and that the device of pulling himself erect on something stable such as furniture and walking holding on was also a useful technique.

Two other techniques used by the well baby also proved useful—walking with arms held above the horizontal as a balancing device, and walking with arms held below the horizontal and used as pistons to pull the body forward.

Finally, the pattern of reproducing "normal" in a child hurt in the cortex took shape as follows. We found it wise to delay the process of walking as long as possible when the child had once reached the level of perfect cross-pattern creeping, since we found that the more he crept, the better his synchronous movements became and the easier it then was to introduce him to walking. When walking had been delayed as long as possible the child was then permitted, when he *insisted* on doing so, to pull himself up into the cruising position on furniture or to walk on his knees if this suited him better. When the child then began to take his first faltering steps without holding on to anything, the team therapy was then directed at making the walking good.

It must be noted here that sometimes the child who is hurt in the cortex is hurt in only one cortex, and man has two cortices—a right and a left cortex. This is of vital importance to man. When a child is hurt in only one side of the cortex, this results in a paralysis of only one side of his body. We found that the longer such a child could be kept creeping, the more likely it was that he would achieve good control of the paralyzed side of his body, whether through maturation of the damaged cortex or even through a transfer of the responsibility for the missing function to the undamaged cortex. (There are many cases on record where an entire hemisphere of the brain has had to be removed surgically—and yet the remaining hemisphere has learned to take over its functions.)

When the child had arrived at the point of being able to take independent steps, even though these steps were poor in nature, then and only then did we begin to prescribe what is now called *cross-pattern walking*. In this method, the child was encouraged to keep his feet a few inches apart, to turn his toes slightly outward, and as he put his left leg forward to bring his right arm forward at the same time and to turn his head slightly to the left. The body is bent laterally at the waist, then as the right leg comes forward, the left arm is also brought forward and at the same time the head is turned slightly to the right.

It seems prudent to point out that this method of walking can hardly be called either the method of Temple Fay or of the team itself. Nor can any of these methods be so described because, as Fay had pointed out long before, they were hardly his methods but instead those of the Good Lord himself. We had simply decided to imitate nature as best we could and to perform these motions as had been intended by nature herself.

We had found that if these patterns were applied rigorously, on a specific schedule, and done with a religious zeal, brain-injured kids improved. If all these things were accomplished and additional central approaches, still to be described, were added, virtually all but the most severely involved youngsters showed marked improvement. We had observed nature and had acted as her Boswell in writing down what we had observed. The approach had paid off.

12.

THE QUESTION OF RECEPTION AND EXPRESSION

May I point out again that the methods described up to this moment, while employing the use of arms and legs and the movement of the head and body in an imitation of what is normal, were not treatments of the arms, legs, head and body but instead of the hurt brain itself. It is vitally important to remember that these methods of patterning were in no sense methods of exercise intended to strengthen arms and legs but instead were *organizing the hurt brain* so that it might perform its own functions. They were therefore, in every sense, a true non-surgical approach to the central problem of the brain itself rather than treatment of the periphery wherein the symptoms lay.

Having found one series of methods for successfully treating the brain-injured child, the question now arose as to whether there were other methods by which he might be successfully treated.

Obviously, in answering this question, the sensible approach would be to find out what other limitations there were in the brain-injured child. In what other ways did he vary from the normal child in his inability to perform?

Here, let me pose to you, the reader, a question that the team had posed to itself a long time before. Suppose you passed a personal friend on the street and said to the friend, "How are you this morning?" If the friend did not answer, what would you assume was the reason for the lack of response? Would you assume that he did not answer because he could not talk—or is it not much more likely that you would assume that he had not heard or seen you?

This illustrates an important question. Can a human being fail to function because of a failure in receiving information, just as he can fail to function because of the inability to express himself? The preceding example would certainly imply that this was true. And yet it was important to note that we had always viewed a failure to function as a failure in the inability to express rather than in the ability to receive. We had said, in essence, that *expression* equaled *function*.

Was it not true that when a human being was unable to bend his knee the world would ask, "What is wrong with his knee or with the muscle in his leg?" We had learned, however, that the failure to move the leg might not exist in the leg itself, but might exist in the front part of the brain or the front part of the spinal cord or anywhere in the motor system, down to the leg itself. Up to now, we had not seriously asked ourselves whether failure to function could occur for reasons that existed outside the motor system.

While we had already added much to our knowledge by observing, as we had, that a failure of function might not exist in the leg itself but might exist within the motor portion of the central nervous system, was it possible that such a failure could exist elsewhere in the central nervous system? This was an important question.

Suppose a child was born deaf. It would follow, would it not, that he would also be unable to talk? Even if he had nothing wrong with his speech mechanism, it would be extremely hard for him to learn to speak words he could not hear.

However, this would be a failure of sensory reception (hearing) rather than a failure of motor output (speech).

If it was true that, in this case, a failure to function might be due to a failure to receive information rather than a failure to express information, then a whole new field of understanding the problems of brain-injured children might open up.

More importantly, if this were true, a whole new field of treatment of the brain-injured child might present itself.

Certainly an investigation of how a human being took in information, as well as how he then expressed himself, seemed in order.

Motor and *sensory* are the medical terms assigned to what we have called expression and reception. Let us review their physiology and workings.

Generally speaking, the back (posterior or dorsal) portion of the brain and spinal cord are responsible for processing all incoming information. These are the sensory or receptive areas of the brain. (See Figure 5.)

Generally speaking, the front (anterior or ventral) portion of the brain and spinal cord are responsible for all outgoing responses. These are called the motor or expressive areas. (See Figure 6.)

This is seen clearly in the names of diseases such as tabes dorsalis (dorsalis meaning back) which is a disease that affects the back of the central nervous system. As a result of tabes, *sensation* is lost, al-

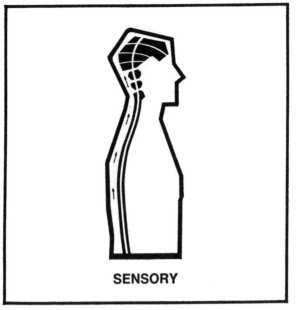

SENSORY

FIGURE 5

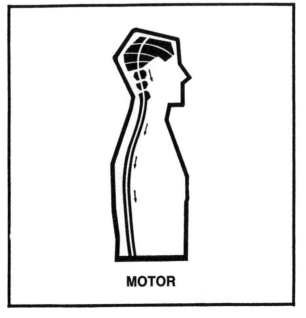

MOTOR

FIGURE 6

though motor abilities in the front of the central nervous system are untouched. (It is highly significant to note here that, although the tabes patient has all his muscles intact and all motor factors are good, he staggers when he walks as does a drunk and eventually does not walk at all, just because he has lost feeling.) This certainly supported our new line of investigation. It might be said, then, that tabes is a receptive, rather than an expressive, disease.

The motor disability is seen clearly in anterior poliomyelitis (infantile paralysis). Polio exists in the *front* of the spinal cord and is therefore called *anterior* poliomyelitis. Polio is a disease that affects only the *motor* system and in no way disturbs sensation or reception. It might be said that it is an *expressive* rather than a *receptive* disease.

If this is true, and we shall verify that it is as we progress, then the formula that we had previously described would have to be expanded, so that instead of saying *expression equals function,* we would have to say *reception plus expression equals function* or, in the words of the medical world, *sensory plus motor equals function.*

What we have stated up to now then is that in order to perform a function, man must be capable not only of commanding his muscles to perform acts, but must, in addition, have certain prior information upon which to base the movements he intends to make. Without such prior information, movement may exist, but it will not be purposeful or functional.

We should examine this view in more detail since understanding it completely is vital to understanding the next method of treating brain-injured children.

What are the sensory or receptive abilities by which man learns—not only about his environment, but indeed about anything at all? While there are many, they can be reduced to five essential areas.

The five ways in which man gains vital information are: (1) seeing, (2) feeling, (3) hearing, (4) smelling, (5) tasting. Many other very important senses such as balance, position sense, etc., exist but can be placed within one or more of the categories above.

A simple experiment will illustrate how dependent we are on our senses. If you should seat yourself before a table upon which has been placed a paper clip, you could pick up the paper clip. It could therefore be said that you have the motor or expressive ability necessary to perform the function of picking up the paper clip.

Let's now see which sensory or receptive factors are employed in picking up the paper clip and eliminate them one at a time until it becomes *impossible* to pick up the paper clip even though the muscles (motor or expressive factors) used in picking it up are still normal and capable of picking up the paper clip—or even something that weighs thousands of times as much.

Before you can perform the motor or expressive act of picking up the paper clip, you must first find out where it is. Obviously, until the paper clip is located it is impossible to pick it up, no matter how strong you might be or how capable. The most commonly used of the receptive senses and probably the one you'd use in picking up the paper clip is vision. You locate the paper clip by seeing it. Then you pick it up. Let us now eliminate vision and see what happens.

If you will now close your eyes and attempt to pick up the paper clip from the table, you will find yourself running your hand over the table to feel for the paper clip. Having eliminated the most commonly used of the senses, vision, you resort to the next of the senses, namely feeling, to locate the paper clip. Having felt it, then you pick it up.

Now let us eliminate both seeing and feeling and see how you will pick up the paper clip. The ideal way to eliminate feel would be to anesthetize the fingers by a local anesthesia but, since this would not be easy as a home experiment, let's do the next best thing, which, while it will not eliminate sensation, will reduce it sufficiently to serve our purposes. If you will now take Scotch tape and completely cover your fingertips down to the first joint—so that no unexposed skin touches the tabletop—we will have enough reduction in feeling for the experiment. If you will now pick up the paper clip with your eyes open, you can still pick up the clip. It will be awkward, since you cannot use your fingernails, but nonetheless, you can still do it.

If you will now close your eyes, we can eliminate both seeing (vision) and feeling (tactility). When you try to pick up the paper clip with eyes closed and feeling gone, you will quickly realize that you cannot and will then begin to make sweeping motions across the table with your fingers. Why do you do this? You realize instinctively that in order to pick up the paper clip, you must first learn its location. You know that there are only five ways to do so—seeing, feeling, hearing, smelling, tasting. We have already made it impossible for you to see (by having you close your eyes) and feel (by anesthetizing your fingertips). You know you can neither smell nor taste the paper clip. You have now resorted to the only remaining sense, that of hearing, to locate the paper clip and you are sweeping your fingers across the table, hoping to *hear* the scraping noise of the paper clip should it become trapped under your sweeping fingers.

Even should this be successful, you will still find it impossible to pick up the clip because you will not *know* when you have been successful. It would little matter if you brought your thumb and forefinger together a thousand times and then lifted them hoping to have within them the paper clip since you would not know if you did indeed have the paper clip.

By this and innumerable other experiments, we can establish that sensation is just as vital to function as motor ability and that if all areas of reception or sensation are destroyed, the human being will be totally unable to function. In accidents involving the spinal cord, any resulting paralysis of the lower limbs may be due more to the loss of sensation *from* those limbs than to the loss of ability to send instructions *to* those limbs.

If one could imagine a human being who had *no* ability to see, feel, hear, taste or smell, one could only imagine the state of death, or of deep coma or of very deep anesthesia. Under such circumstances, although a human being might have a brain of the rarest genius, of what value would it be?

If a genius were unable to receive any of the five sensations, how could he even verify the fact that he was alive? He could not pinch himself to prove that he was alive, because he couldn't feel it even if he did pinch himself. He could not cry aloud, for even if he did he could not hear himself to verify that he had cried. He could not look to verify the existence of his body, for he could not see. He could not so much as smell or taste himself.

Experiments have been performed on extremely healthy young men who for periods of time volunteered to be isolated in total silence and darkness with all other factors reduced as much as possible without inducing unconsciousness. Although only a few of the five senses were totally eliminated, in a few hours these healthy young men were almost totally disoriented as to time and space and were not able to say how long they had been maintained in this state or what had happened during that time.

From these and hundreds of other experiments we may conclude that man can only be totally complete to the degree that he has his receptive factors intact.

We may further conclude that if all of a man's receptive factors were removed, a deathlike state would follow and remain at least until they were returned.

If, between these two extremes, man's faculties for learning are removed one at a time, we will reduce his ability to function.

We could therefore conclude very positively that it was *essential* to man's function that he have sensory intake, or reception.

Helen Keller's fame was not due essentially to the fact of her accomplishments, it was due to what she accomplished *without* two of her vital receptive qualities, seeing and hearing. The world has long recognized the tremendous handicap that such losses bring about.

It soon became clear that brain-injured children are usually deficient in at least some of their receptor functions. Children whose problem is a result of Rh incompatibility are sometimes deaf, others are sometimes blind, and most brain-injured children have reduced ability to feel. We now examined the rest of them carefully through new and more skilled eyes to see to what extent the brain injury might have caused sensory problems as well as motor problems, because we now knew that they were equally vital to function.

It was clearly important never to forget for a moment that there are: (1) sensory (receptive) pathways which bring information into the brain, and (2) motor (expressive) pathways through which the brain reacts by commanding motor responses based on the information it has received.

Fay had taught us that all incoming sensory pathways are a one-way road into the brain and are incapable of carrying an outgoing message, while all outgoing motor pathways were equally one-way and are incapable of carrying a message into the brain. This was a long-recognized and well-known fact of neurology, but the world's failure to apply it in the diagnosis of the symptoms of brain injury explained in part exactly why the conventional rehabilitation techniques were so ineffective. Classical methods had tried to treat the brain-injured patient in purely motor terms. The results of that motor-oriented treatment had been that whatever information had managed to reach the brain had been both accidental and incidental.

Dr. Fay, virtually alone in medicine, had been fascinated by the work of that great mathematical genius Norbert Wiener, and had not only understood Wiener's book *Cybernetics* but had also understood its implications for human beings—most especially brain-injured human beings. He had insisted that I read and understand it as well.

It was clear that the human brain, like Dr. Wiener's self-regulating systems, operated like a cybernetic loop—and a superb one.

The normal cybernetic functioning of the brain is completely dependent upon the integrity of all of these pathways. The *total* destruction of all motor *or* all sensory pathways will result in *total* lack of functional performance of the human being. The *partial* destruction of one or the other will result in *partial* lack of functional performance.

It is also depressingly clear that such lack of function will continue until the former specific pathways are restored to function or until new pathways are established that are capable of completing the total loop.

In human beings this loop, which begins in the environment, follows sensory pathways to the brain and motor pathways from the brain back to the environment. (See Figure 7.)

All efforts in treatment of the brain-injured child would therefore have to be directed toward locating the break and closing the circuit.

Could we find procedures to locate the break and thereafter to close the circuit? We would have to if we were to solve the problems of our brain-injured children.

But how?

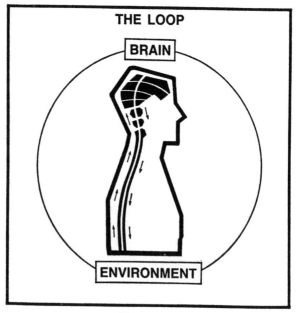

FIGURE 7

13.

THE INSTITUTES ARE BORN

Finding the break in the circuit was only one of innumerable problems which faced us. By now we had organizational problems, too.

While I would be reluctant to say that I believe in miracles in the old-fashioned religious sense, I must say that there have been some periods of time during which I have felt that I was being shoved about by forces beyond my control. One such period began in the last half of 1954.

As the team had continued to grow during the early 1950s it had been necessary that some structure emerge to make functioning possible.

We had agreed years before to continue to see Dr. Fay's patients in the nursing home into which Dr. Fay's Neurophysical Rehabilitation Center had been converted. The original idea had been that we would see his post-operative patients until they had all been discharged from the nursing home. These patients ran the gamut of adult brain-injured patients—from stroke patients to Parkinson's disease—and included many relatively rare neurological disorders. Seeing such patients meant that after Dr. Fay had operated on them I would be responsible for their post-operative rehabilitation.

We had expected our patient population in the nursing home to decline as our patients were discharged and as aged patients coming for domiciliary care took their place, freeing us to spend *all* of our time in our offices seeing patients together.

That is not what happened. After an initial falling off of patients as anticipated, new patients began to seek admission to the nursing home not as a domiciliary care unit but, instead, to receive the treatment services of our team. The United Cerebral Palsy Association also began sending us children as patients. (By this time the team consisted of Dr. Fay as the neurosurgeon, my brother as the physiatrist, Carl Delacato as the psychologist, and me as a sort of director of rehabilitation services since by this time I had several physical

therapists and an occupational therapist working for me. Claude
Cheek served as speech therapist.)

What had happened was that we had grown into a rehabilitation
center, one of the earliest in the country.

We had many problems, and as the director, these problems
weighed heavily on me. In the first place, the buildings and grounds
were inadequate to the task before us. Since most of the buildings
and ground belonged to the nursing home, we could not make the
changes we wished, and since the objective of the nursing home and
its owners was to make money rather than to solve problems, which
was their right, we found ourselves frustrated in our attempts to do
research or to do teaching.

We were beginning to receive requests from physicians and therapists, here and abroad, who wished to visit our "institute" to study
the work we were doing. We had neither time, money nor facility
to do any such teaching.

What was needed was crystal clear, but how to come by it was far
less clear. What was needed was a non-profit organization, organized
for the purpose of research, training and treatment in the field of
brain-injured patients. It should be organized along the lines of a
typical hospital or university. Such an organization should have buildings, grounds and staff adequate to treat inpatients, to conduct clinical research and to teach other professional people what we were
doing, how we were doing it and why we were doing it.

A reasonably large amount of ground would be required, certainly
no less than several acres, and in Chestnut Hill land sold by the foot.
Certainly the ground would cost $25,000.

Also needed would be a minimum of forty beds plus treatment
areas, etc. In those days a rule of thumb for the cost of building patient beds was $10,000 per bed, which meant that building would
cost about a half million dollars.

In addition, a minimum staff of about ten first-rate professional
people would be needed, as well as about ten service people, such
as cooks, laundress, plant engineer, etc. By the most stringent
economies salaries could not fail to be less than $150,000 per year.

Food, heat, electricity, telephones, etc., would surely cost no less
than a hundred thousand dollars for the first year.

In short, we would need close to a million dollars just to get
started.

Dr. Fay, although he could command huge surgical fees, seldom
did, and he had not yet recovered from the financial disaster of The

Neurophysical Rehabilitation Center. Bob, Carl and Claude were even younger than I and recently out of school. That left me, and everyone looked to me for a solution. I needed a million dollars and I knew where I could get about forty-three dollars.

It was just about then that the events began which led me to feel that I was being pushed around by forces outside my control.

It was the very day when I had decided that there was simply no way to solve the problem when the first thing happened. Betty Marsh came to see me. Betty Marsh was a very nice middle-aged, red-headed, Irish practical nurse who worked for the nursing home and who would often bring patients over to my office in wheel chairs when I called for them. Although she and I had often exchanged pleasantries, I hadn't remembered her name. Although she was a registered practical nurse, what she had to say to me was as impractical as anything I had ever heard—and strangely insightful.

She had, she said, been watching the results of the work in the Rehabilitation Center and thought it was the most kind work she had ever seen. She thought that if human beings could be that kind to each other perhaps there was some hope for us all. She had noticed how tremendously busy I was and lately she had felt that perhaps I had not been entirely happy with the circumstances at the nursing home.

Then she dropped her bomb. She felt, she said, that it was very important to the people of the world that my work be continued. While she knew nothing of the situation, she wanted me to know that she had lived very carefully all of her life and that she had saved up six thousand dollars and that these six thousand dollars were in the bank and that I could have them anytime I wanted them, and I could pay them back if I was ever able to do so. There would, she announced, be no paper signing of any kind (a process she mistrusted) and no interest paying, which took all the good out of a good thing.

I mumbled my appreciation of her kind thought and sat stunned as she blithely took her departure pushing her now empty wheel chair.

What the devil did it mean?

How had she guessed that a problem even existed?

Why in the name of everything sensible would this single little woman without security of any kind offer me her lifetime savings when I was almost a stranger to her?

What in hell was her name?

While I had not the slightest intention of accepting her offer, I was totally overcome by her unbelievable generosity to a man who didn't even know her name. I was seething with conflicting emotions.

On one hand her extremely strange insight and incredible generosity had moved me close to tears. On the other hand she also made me feel extremely selfish and rather cowardly and, in a way, unworthy of the work I was doing. I had been overwhelmed by the need for hundreds of thousands of dollars and had decided to give up such an impossible dream as being out of the question. Yet it was obvious to me that six thousand dollars must represent more money to her than hundreds of thousands of dollars did to me. Yet she had offered it all. While it was unquestionably true that six thousand dollars was more money to her than hundreds of thousands were to me, it was also true that those sums of money had less worth to her than they had to me. I was ashamed.

I got through my work that day in a mechanical way, which was not characteristic, but I was mightily distracted by what had happened. I was not even given the rest of the day to recover.

As I finished work, Mae Blackburn proposed that we sit awhile and talk.

Mae had been a yeomanette in the U. S. Navy in World War I and also, I had been told, a crack secretary. I had seen Mae first as a patient three or four years earlier. She weighed eighty-eight pounds, was a few years older than my mother and looked old enough to be my grandmother.

Mae's problem needed no psychiatrist to understand. Mae was in her early sixties but she was very young at heart. Her husband had died and so had most of her friends, and those that hadn't had grown old more willingly than Mae. Her son was married and gone and Mae was alone. Mae had not taken care of herself and when I saw her first she had not the strength to walk. Good food, regular hours, no parties and a sensible program of exercise had set her right in a few months and she had been discharged as well. Six months later she was back and the entire process was repeated. Then she came back for the third time.

It was then that I had put into effect a little scheme that backfired. I had up to that time been my own secretary (I had the virtue of being both cheap and careful.) When Mae Blackburn had returned for the third time, painfully thin, exhausted and so shaky that she could not light her own cigarette, I had proposed that perhaps she could help me by typing a letter or two. Although the thought obviously frightened her, she had agreed to try. Her letters were absolutely terrible in the beginning, and I would take them home at night and retype them with two fingers. Since that is what I would have had to do anyway, there was no extra work for me and it was clearly good for her. Very quickly her letters improved until they were perfect and so, too, was she. It was obviously time for her to be discharged since she no longer needed me. My clever game had backfired, however, because now *I* needed *her*.

So Mae had gone to work for me at a terribly inadequate salary to become my secretary, my bookkeeper, my second mother, my boss and my friend.

I sat on the desk and listened in stupefaction while Mae offered me *her* life savings. Since Mae got a tiny salary, she only had three thousand dollars saved, but it was mine.

I saw a plot of some sort and accused her of collaborating with what's-her-name, the redheaded Irish nurse. She obviously did not know what I was talking about, but she did know that the redheaded Irish nurse was named Betty Marsh. I told her with wonder what had happened that morning. She had known nothing about it, but she saw nothing unusual in the story since she also thought the work was kind and wonderful. She thought everyone ought to help. She was surprised that everyone hadn't offered to help, and the fact that no one knew about the problem did not seem to her a good reason not to help. Nobody had told her and Marshy about it, but they knew, didn't they? I agreed in a trancelike way that they did.

Even today I find it difficult to believe my own story, and perhaps I would find it harder to believe, now that many more years have passed, if I did not daily look out my office window across the lovely green lawn to the Mae Blackburn Building. It helps me to remember that amazing woman. It also helps me to remember Betty Marsh when I look out my office window toward the Mae Blackburn Building because my office itself is in the Betty Marsh Building.

Mae Blackburn had insisted also, in addition to lending me the three thousand dollars, that she could, would and insisted on working free in whatever the "new place" was.

I had difficulty sleeping that night because I did not know what the "new place" was. I had the feeling I was getting pushed around by factors beyond my control. It is a feeling I have had many, many times since, and I have learned to relax and not resist even when I do not entirely understand.

Both of these women, I thought that night, are far older than I.

They have no security at all. Yet through some prescience which I did not understand they had both insisted on giving everything they had. What of me? What was everything I had? Was I willing to give it?

Well, I had my equipment and all the furniture in my large house. All of that could be donated to be used in the "new place," whatever that meant. That was worth nine or ten thousand dollars.

Then there was the house itself. Although a large mortgage still remained, I could sell it and realize fourteen thousand dollars and that also could be donated.

Altogether it sounded to me as if I could scrape up about thirty-two thousand dollars. Only a drop in the bucket. It couldn't be done, and so I would tell those two crazy women tomorrow. *How* could I tell them that? They simply wouldn't understand.

Maybe though, with Mae's idea of working free . . . Suppose all the professional people worked free for awhile until we got going? I got out of bed and got pencil and paper.

Suppose by some miracle we had the place in which to work. Maybe we could rent it or something. Could we then make it work? If there were a place to work we might by a miracle make it for a couple of months if we had forty thousand dollars instead of thirty-two.

Two nights later Mr. Massingham, my father-in-law, offered me eight thousand dollars. It was obvious how he knew about the problem. I had told him—but without having the foggiest notion that he might help to solve it. Both he and Mom had been very poor as children in England and although Dad had done well in America he had been unable to forget about his childhood poverty and was extremely cautious with money. He had simply not occurred to me as a source of money.

Dr. Fay agreed to work free. So also did my brother. So, of course, did my wife.

It was then that Miss Galbraith asked to see me. By now I was used to people asking to see me, and I went half expecting her to offer help. Libbeth Galbraith was a patient. She was a fifty-year-old brain-injured kid with the problem that most people call cerebral palsy. These are the people who, when they are severe, are in constant writhing motion. These are the people who look so awful (when they are severe). Most people assume them to be mentally retarded when in truth they are smart, smart, smart.

Libbeth was unlike the severe athetoid cerebral palsy type in that she did not writhe, although she could not walk, but she was like all other athetoids in that she was smart, smart, smart. She was also most insightful. Although she and I spent a part of every day getting her out of her wheel chair and teaching her to walk for the first time in fifty years, we had never discussed my problem.

This night we did. We drove to Fairmount Park and as we drove Libbeth talked. She believed I should go have a talk with her brother-in-law, A. Vinton Clarke, and her sister, Helen Clarke.

I had only met Mr. Clarke once before in my life and that most casually. I was sure he would not even remember me, and when I called to make an appointment this proved to be true. He did not remember me. Nonetheless, he invited me to his house the following evening.

He listened carefully as I told him of our hopes and dreams. Taking a deep breath, I told him that to get started I believed I needed about twenty-five thousand dollars. He slowly shook his head no. You will need, he told me, more like eighty thousand dollars. Having said so, he handed me a check for eighty thousand dollars. Although I had never so much as seen that much money and although I was extremely grateful, I was no longer surprised.

Neither was I surprised when I found the "new place." It was a superb estate in Chestnut Hill. There were eight acres in that original site and two superb buildings as well as lovely greenhouses and a barn. There were more than a quarter of a million dollars' worth of beautiful trees and bushes. The place was obviously worth millions of dollars and was absolutely ideal for our purposes. I wasn't surprised that I had found the ideal place for us.

I wasn't even surprised when I called the agent to find out how much the estate would cost. The firm sale price was exactly eighty thousand dollars.

What do you think of that for being pushed around?

Aside from my work, the only friends I had were military friends. I had, after the war, believed that the world was far from safe and I had remained in the active reserve. I had joined Philadelphia's ancient 111th Infantry Regiment of the Pennsylvania National Guard. The commander of that regiment was Col. Jay Cooke, an outstanding Philadelphian whose great-grandfather, Jay Cooke, had financed the Civil War for the Union.

It was he who had promoted me to captain when I had joined the regiment, and it was his former estate which we bought. Since I had been his guest there I had known about it. He had lived there with his wife and two daughters, and when he had found himself alone with a huge staff of servants after the death of his wife and the marriage of his daughters he had offered the place for auction. The very wealthy man who had bought it had realized quickly that even a wealthy man could not afford to support such an estate, and he sold it to us.

Jay Cooke came to serve as a member of the board of directors of the "new place" until the day of his death in 1963.

On July 22, 1955, after months of work, the Honorable Judge William F. Dannehower of the Court of Common Pleas of Montgomery County, Pennsylvania, decreed that The Rehabilitation Center at Philadelphia be approved as a non-profit corporation.

The directors were Glenn Doman, Robert Doman, Frank D. McCormick (a military friend), Temple Fay, Claude Cheek, and Martin Palmer.

Thomas R. White, Jr. (a prominent Philadelphia attorney and a senior officer of my regiment) was to serve The Institute as attorney until his death years later. He did so without pay.

Robert Magee, one of my oldest and closest friends, had served as the first president of the board of governors.

Major General Arthur D. Kemp served as a member of the board of governors from the day of that body's inception, and later as its president, until its service was completed many years later.

Bob Magee's wife, Doris, served several terms as president of the women's board and still remains an active part of that active group.

They served, all of them, because they were personal friends and for the love of the children, and this they found reward enough.

The Rehabilitation Center at Philadelphia would later change its name to The Institutes for the Achievement of Human Potential.

So—with a number of shoves—The Institutes for the Achievement of Human Potential were born—and just in time.

14.

SENSATION AND ITS IMPORTANCE TO MOVEMENT

We have noted that without incoming (sensory or receptive) factors an otherwise well adult human brain will fail to function in even so simple a process as picking up a paper clip. It can be imagined what such receptive losses would mean to the much more complex acts of walking and talking in a brain-injured child who had *never known about such things in the first place.*

We now had to determine where the brain-injured children had suffered such losses, and to what degree. If they had such losses, we then had to determine whether anything could be done about this *since such losses by themselves could prevent not only walking and talking but even far simpler acts.*

We had determined that there are five human receptive abilities that make it possible for a human to obtain information of any kind, from the most complex sort (understanding nuclear physics) to the most simple sort (understanding that the radiator is burning the leg which is lying against it). The five receptive areas in man are: (1) seeing, (2) feeling, (3) hearing, (4) smelling, (5) tasting.

Smelling and tasting are essentially recessive characteristics in man, and our dogs are more skilled in them than we are. For well adults these characteristics are essentially pleasure seeking. They are extremely important to certain specialists, such as wine tasters and perfume sniffers. Adults derive most of their operating information from the other three.

This chapter will deal with seeing, hearing and feeling.

We had begun to feel that we understood how a child learns to see, hear and feel in broad terms, and we had as yet spent only a little time on how he learns to smell and taste.

VISION

We again went first to well children to study how they learned to see, and we found that they progressed through four important stages, which, generally speaking, corresponded to the four stages we had seen in mobility, stages that were normally completed by the age of twelve to eighteen months. We were struck with this coincidence, and later events proved that we were wise to have noted what would prove to be a most important relationship.

Much ingenuity was required to test these children and to determine what they saw since visual testing is usually based on the patient's verbal responses to what he sees. None of the children under one year of age could answer such questions, and many of the brain-injured children over one year of age had speech problems. New methods had to be developed and new equipment designed with which we could come to a determination of what a child saw without asking him to answer questions. This was not easy, and even the methods we developed did not tell us all we wanted to know. Nonetheless, we learned a good many things.

The four stages through which well children passed in learning to see were as follows:

Stage 1—In the days that immediately followed birth a child reacted reflexively to light and to darkness. This is called a light reflex. It was not safe to say that he perceived light or that he understood light, for such appreciation is impossible until higher stages come into play. His reaction was completely reflex in nature. When light fell on his eye the pupil constricted, when the light was removed the pupil dilated.

Stage 2—During this stage, the well baby began to gain outline perception and to differentiate varying degrees of light; that is to say, he could see a human silhouette if the person were outlined against the light, and he would respond to less bright light shined toward his face. He could follow a human being about the room with his eyes if that person were outlined against a light.

Stage 3—During this stage he began to see detail when a light was thrown on an object itself and to appreciate the differences in detail of such an object. He could now see an object within a larger configuration. Vision took on added meaning. (He could differentiate the buttons on mother's blouse from the blouse itself.)

Stage 4—During this stage, which began at about one year of age and which would not be complete in all its human detail until almost eight years of age, many, many important things took place. Principal among these was the characteristic called *stereopsis* or depth perception. In the human being this is another function of the cortex. (Here again was reconfirmation of our original ideas.) This cortical function of stereopsis did not begin until myelination had begun to take place in the cortex at about one year of life. (Myelination is the process by which a soft, white, fatty substance called *myelin* encases the axon or tail of certain neurons [nerve cells], thus making them able to function.)

We came to realize that a very high percentage of brain-injured children have visual problems; in fact, we were daily becoming more convinced that virtually all brain-injured children had some visual problem despite the fact that some had eyes that appeared to be normal to external examination and showed no obvious signs of visual deficiencies.

We have also seen many seriously injured children who did not react, either consciously or reflexively, even to a strong light shining in their eyes. This is blindness. For many years we felt that this was a situation where we could do nothing other than pray, for if a child was blind, what was there to do? But as years went by, we began to see a startling phenomenon which we did not even attempt to explain, other than to feel that it was a most fortunate coincidence. Many of the children who in the beginning appeared to be blind began to gain small amounts of vision. Others who had had small amounts of vision began to gain greater amounts of vision. This was exceedingly strange since we were doing nothing whatsoever that we considered to be in the nature of visual treatment.

As more children began to gain ground visually, it became necessary to ask whether this was actually a coincidence or was a result of something that was happening to the children.

Up to this time we had not kept progress notes on children's vision but had only examined them thoroughly at the beginning of their treatment period, since we viewed vision as a static affair—something that would not improve. Now we began to keep progress notes.

We began to see that this visual gain was more than coincidence because it was apparent that the children who were making visual gains were the same children who were making gains in mobility. If treatment stopped for any reason and mobility progress stopped, visual progress also stopped. When treatment was again resumed and mobility again improved, we began again to see visual progress. What was making these visual gains occur?

As I think I have demonstrated repeatedly in this book, hindsight always checks out at 20/20. Looking back now, these startling facts are understandable. Indeed, it is extremely ironic that, in light of the views that the group held, we should have been surprised to see progress in visual areas. It is surprising that people who had devoted so much of their lives to establishing the fact that brain injury lies within the brain did not see this point. We ourselves had said repeatedly: If the problem lies within the brain, it will do no good to treat the elbows, nose, ears and eyes, where only the symptoms of the problems exist.

We ourselves had fallen into the very trap we had sometimes criticized others for falling into. We had been thinking of blindness as a problem of the eyes instead of a symptom of a problem within the brain. Indeed, why should it be strange that vision improved if we were, in fact, as we intended to do, treating the brain itself? If, in fact, the difficulty that caused the paralysis of the leg existed within the brain as we said it did, then might not the difficulty that caused the visual problem also exist within the brain itself? Here was a question of tremendous import.

Why should such a very high percentage of the brain-injured have visual problems of great magnitude? Did we have a right to suspect that the children who were brain-injured also had had something else happen to their eyes which gave them visual problems? This hardly seemed likely. Was it not much more likely that the children who had brain injury were having visual problems due to the brain injury itself? Could we not say that if a problem existed within the brain then the chances were good that a brain-injured child would also have difficulty seeing for the same reason that he had difficulty moving a leg or an arm?

After all, there was plenty of evidence that a human being could have a visual problem that did not exist in the eye itself. He could, and very frequently did. We repeatedly had seen visual problems in brain-injured adults following a stroke. We knew of the visual problems that beset the adult brain in Parkinson's disease. We know of the visual problems that could beset an adult when his adult brain was hurt in an automobile or a diving accident.

We were not observing some strange miracle when we saw vision restored in brain-injured children, but rather we were observing the only logical course we could expect if, indeed, we were treating a brain rather than an elbow or an eye.

We turned with renewed energy to probing the visual problems such children demonstrate.

In brief, we found that those children had all of the visual problems that confronted the brain-injured adult.

We saw in these children the exact same sort of vision defects that we saw in adult stroke patients. Some of these children saw nothing to the left of the nose or nothing to the right of the nose or nothing above the horizontal or nothing below the horizontal. Some had the visual problem of constricted fields in which the entire cone of a child's vision was greatly diminished, permitting little vision to the sides, top and bottom.

We also detected scotomas (blank spots) in the vision of some of these children, although these were hard to detect since the children were not capable of telling us about their visual problems and such sophisticated testing as was necessary to determine the presence of a scotoma was difficult to perform.

Some of the children could see at near point (within arm's length) but could not see at far point (beyond arm's length); in others this was reversed. Some children could see fairly well but could not detect detail.

Most common of all, we found problems of fusion in our children. These problems were very easy to detect since they were generally accompanied by an easy-to-see strabismus.

The word strabismus, you will remember, is the medical term for what is generally called either cross-eye or walleye, or sometimes a squint. If one eye turns in, this is called a *convergent unilateral strabismus.* If one eye turns outward, this is called a *divergent unilateral strabismus.* If one eye turns upward, this is called a *superior unilateral strabismus.* If one eye turns downward, it is called an *inferior unilateral strabismus.* If both eyes do so, the unilateral is simply changed to bilateral so that if we saw a child who was cross-eyed in both eyes, this child would be recorded as having a *convergent bilateral strabismus.*

These problems are extremely common. Particularly is this so in those children who have problems in the midbrain starting at or before birth. While a marked strabismus is rather easy to detect, even by the least initiated person, a very small strabismus is not and requires careful examination of the eyes. This examination, however, can be performed by parents themselves simply by observation of the child's eyes and the way they move.

If a child has a strabismus, it is quite obvious that he cannot have fused vision since to have fused vision, the eyes must converge on the object being seen. Occasionally one sees a child who has a strabismus habitually, until such time as he looks specifically at an object, at which time the strabismus may disappear and he may actually see that object in proper depth. If a child has a strabismus that is always present, or if he has a strabismus that alternates from eye to eye, he obviously cannot see in depth.

What, then, does the child see who does have a strabismus? We know that he does not see in depth. It is possible also that he actually sees two different visual images. When this is the case, what the child is seeing is called *diplopia*.

Let us say that a child has a right convergent strabismus, that is to say that his left eye looks at the object which he intends to look at, while the right crosses over that axis of vision to see something else. The left eye might therefore be looking at a lamp in front of the child while the right eye is actually seeing a scene far to the child's left.

Is there an alternative to a child seeing two images if the eyes are in fact seeing two different scenes? Yes, there is; it is most likely that if the strabismus is severe, the child will learn very quickly to ignore entirely one visual image. He learns to "look at" (pay attention to) only one of the images, or only one at a time. This process is called *cortical suppression*.

The methods we have since developed to get maximal visual abilities out of a child will be described in a future book, but, in summary, these things can now be recorded. Visual problems in a brain-injured child should not be considered surprising since the visual tracts run the length of the brain from the eye to the occipital area in the back of the head itself. It is easy to see how many different kinds of brain injury can affect this visual pathway, thus creating a visual problem that does not exist in the eye itself but exists somewhere between the eye and the back of the brain.

The team also came to realize that many secondary involvements might occur as a result of brain injury. It would be necessary to treat also these secondary things that had happened as a result of the inactivity brought about by the brain injury. In other words, in the case of restored vision, the team sometimes had to teach the child how to use that new visual capacity.

We now began to ask ourselves an extremely interesting question. Was it possible to treat the brain for one missing function *without* seeing results in all areas? We asked ourselves a question that was more amusing than realistic. Suppose a parent came to us with a brain-injured child saying, "I should like you to make my child walk, but I do not want him to see."

The moral question aside, could we have accomplished this? Could we have hoped to develop movement and walking in this brain-injured child without at the same time achieving results in vision if both were the result of the same injury? It hardly seemed likely.

It would not be fair to leave this section on vision without pointing out one visual problem which we find in brain-injured children but do not find in adults who were hurt in later life. It is a serious handicap. The adult who sustains an injury that creates for him a visual problem has one tremendous advantage: He *has* known what the world looks like. He knows what seeing is. The brain-injured child has no such advantage.

FEELING

There is no more important system for the preservation of life than the sensory mechanism we call feeling. Without this tactile mechanism we would exist in constant danger of the destruction of life itself. By feeling, we are warned of the dangers that threaten us. The quadriplegic patient who has lost the ability to feel from the neck down as a result of a severely damaged spinal cord may sit with his leg against a radiator and not be aware of the fact that his leg is burning until he actually smells the burning flesh, since in him the sense of smell is intact, while tactility is not.

Suppose that we did not have the pain which we frequently complain so bitterly about. If there were no pain, how would one ever know that appendicitis existed? It is the pain that leads us to perform the laboratory tests which so frequently confirm the presence of the inflammation. Without such pain it is quite likely that few human beings would ever be operated on for appendicitis. They would instead die of the unchecked disease.

Where, in the human, does feeling exist? It would almost be easier to answer the question, where does it not exist? At least in the external covering of the body it exists virtually everywhere, and if you were to close your eyes and ask someone else to touch you somewhere on your body, you could detect this touch even if it were your

hair he touched, since even the movement of the hair would make
itself felt on the scalp.

We wanted first to look at how feeling or tactile sensation develops
in the well child up to one year of age, as we had long since learned
was the proper course. We found again a fact that was most interesting to us: In normal children the area of feeling developed in four
stages and these four stages again paralleled the four stages we had
seen in mobility and in vision. These four stages are:

Stage one, which exists essentially during the first month of life,
has primarily to do with those sensations that are of the most basic
and primitive sort. These sensations are entirely reflex in nature. They
are skin reflexes, which are present at birth and which do not require
decision from the brain at all. These reflex reactions go only through
the sensory pathway to the spinal cord and directly from the spinal
cord back through the motor pathway to the muscular system. An example of this is the Babinski reflex. Here the examiner scrapes a point
such as a key along the bottom of the infant's foot. In the normal infant the toes will turn upward and fan out (a positive Babinski). This
is normal in an infant but abnormal in a well adult. In a well adult the
toes will turn downward and come together (a negative Babinski).

Stage two exists from about four weeks of life up to several months,
during which time the child responds to stimuli from outside the body.
However, these stimuli, to affect the child, have to be of a vital nature
and must actually threaten the child's existence. He responds during
this stage of his life to vital stimuli, to vital feeling, to feeling that,
if continued, would actually threaten life itself, such as a pin stick
or extreme pain of any kind. This period could be called the period
of vital sensation. His response is to withdraw from the pain and to
cry for help.

Stage three, which comes fully into play by about seven months
of age, is the stage of the child's existence in which he comes to understand the so-called gnostic sensations, sensations that are less
strong than the vital sensations that might threaten life. During this
period of time the well child is able to identify things as being not
merely hot but also warm, not merely cold but also cool, not merely
very painful but also uncomfortable. The child now reacts to con-
tentment because of pleasant stimuli, such as dry diapers, etc., and
reacts unpleasantly to those things that might be uncomfortable, such
as wet diapers (which he is now able to recognize). Also during this
period of time a factor very vital to his walking begins—the beginning of balance. Balance is a very important product of sensation.

It draws from all of the three basic sensory areas but has important ramifications in tactile sensation itself. During this period of life the child's feeling varies a great deal, and if there are areas in which he is undersensitive, there are also areas in which he is oversensitive to certain kinds of stimuli.

The fourth stage begins at approximately one year. During this period, which is the beginning of the development of the cortex, the child begins to develop stereognosis, which is the tactile equivalent of stereopsis (depth perception). By feeling an object between his fingers he can identify it in remarkable detail and he begins to appreciate the fact that objects felt have depth just as do those objects that can be "felt" with the eyes. His sense of feeling now becomes highly discriminative. He acquires, during this period, the heightened sense of balance necessary to the upright or walking position. He acquires two-point discrimination and certain other very advanced tactile qualities.

In examining our children, we came to the conclusion, as we had with vision, that it was a rare brain-injured child who did not have some problem in some area of sensation. Sometimes the problem was as small as not being able to distinguish mildly warm from mildly cool, even though the ability to differentiate between hot and cold might be present. Sometimes the problem was so severe that the child was virtually devoid of sensation and was in as much danger, due to this factor, as was the quadriplegic. The brain-injured child was also frequently oversensitive, and this was often as large a problem as having too little sensitivity.

It was interesting to note that until a well child reached the age of five or six, even he did not have as good sensation, in some ways, as the adult. Perhaps you have had the experience of having your own head butted by a small child's—resulting in a good deal of pain in your head and a good deal of delight on the part of the child who is not disturbed by the tremendous blow.

We frequently saw brain-injured children who could lie, with no apparent discomfort, on top of a large object on the floor, such as a plastic toy. We drew the conclusion that they did not feel the object. We concluded that many of the brain-injured children were not even aware that their arms and legs actually belonged to them or had any connection with their bodies. If a child could be unaware that his legs were his, he could hardly be expected to move these legs in a manner that would teach him to crawl, to creep and to walk.

Again, as with vision, we came to the conclusion that the problems did not truly exist in the arms and legs of the children but rather existed in that portion of the spinal cord or nervous system that was responsible for all incoming information.

These children were handicapped, indeed, since the child who did not gain information could not possibly function. A child could not put out functional movement if he did not first take in the information on which the functional activities were based. (You will remember your own experience with the paper clip.)

Finding ways of treating this problem within the brain itself was the next assignment we gave ourselves, and over a period of many years sensory techniques have been developed which, while they are applied to arms, legs and body, are not expected to affect the arms, legs and body directly, but instead are a method of giving information to an injured brain relative to where its arms and legs *are*.

HEARING

The brain-injured child had problems in hearing, also.

We learned rather quickly that auditory acuity was not the most important element of hearing just as visual acuity was not the most important part of seeing. While complete lack of auditory acuity (deafness) was often present in our children, it was much more common to find children who could hear but could not hear in a way that permitted them to interpret what they heard.

When we measured how a child learns to hear and what he understands from what he hears, we could define the same four stages we had seen in the other areas.

Stage one, immediately following birth, we found, is the period when what a child takes in through his ears is of a purely reflex nature. When a loud noise occurs he jumps in what is called a *startle reflex*. This implies no fright or fear on the part of the child, nor does it demonstrate an understanding of what he hears. It is a simple reflex activity.

Stage two begins when a sudden loud noise can be interpreted by the child as a possible threat to his life. Now, in addition to being startled, he cries. It might be said that he is crying for help in response to what could be a threat to his life.

Stage three occurs when the child begins to understand the meaning of sounds. Words do not yet have significance at this stage, but the tone of mother's voice is highly significant. If mother scolds, baby cries even though he does not understand her words. This is the stage of meaningful sound.

Stage four again occurs between a year and eighteen months of life, and again it deals with a depth factor. This time it has to do with the depth of meaning of words themselves. By now the baby understands not only the meaning of sound but also the meaning of words themselves.

While at this time it would appear that hearing problems are less common and perhaps even less important than those problems existing in the areas of vision and of feeling, nonetheless, it is quite true that such problems do exist, and there is reason to suspect that there are aberrations in hearing not only among some specific groups of children who are frequently deaf (such as those who are the result of incompatible Rh factors) but also among those children and adults who are hurt in the midbrain.

We know that those people hurt in midbrain, such as the children who are described as having athetoid cerebral palsy, frequently have a marked startle reflex; that is to say, they respond with huge jumps and body stiffening to sudden noises. These patients also frequently complain that certain sounds are actually painful to their ears—painful, not simply undesirable or uncomfortable. We have come to realize that in Parkinson's disease there is an oversensitivity of hearing which makes these patients talk lower since it is not necessary to, as they put it, "shout." We also know that in injuries resulting from certain kinds of accidents, such as automobile accidents, the patient frequently talks far too loudly. These three abnormalities in hearing can all be related to the same area of brain even though they appear to be very unlike each other.

Thus, as the clouds of mystery that hid the truth from us were gradually being blown away by the fresh and stimulating winds of new knowledge, one could see that sensory intake was not only as important to human function as was motor ability, but that all motor ability was *based on* sensory intake.

It was now clear that there could be four degrees of sensory problems (in visual, auditory or tactile terms) in the brain-injured child. These were:

1. The total absence of visual, auditory or tactile intake (blindness, deafness, insensateness). These were disastrous to the brain-injured child if permitted to continue.

2. Too little visual, auditory or tactile intake (hard of seeing, hard

of hearing, hard of feeling). These were overwhelming handicaps to the brain-injured child if permitted to remain.

3. Too much visual, auditory and tactile intake (oversensitive reception of such stimuli). This was equally overwhelming.

4. Chaotic visual, auditory or tactile intake (receiving distorted visual, auditory or tactile information as, for example, the visual information received by the child with strabismus). This could likewise be discouraging, disconcerting or frightening.

It was becoming daily more clear, as we saw more and more severely brain-injured children, that one or many of these problems was usually in the picture, though the degree of disability could range from the almost imperceptible to total. It was rare that a hurt kid didn't have some of them.

What was more, as we began to make more gains in mobility, we also saw more gains in visual, auditory and tactile areas. There seemed to be some connection, even if we couldn't yet quite explain it.

If true dawn had not yet arrived, perhaps it could be said that first light was upon us and that silhouettes of the shapes of tomorrow's formulations could be dimly seen. However indistinct the picture, at least it seemed to be taking shape.

15.

BREATHING

The matter of breathing and the manner in which the brain-injured child breathes are also terribly important—and a most interesting story.

It is breathing that supplies the oxygen to the brain which is vital to the well human being and which is at least as vital to the brain-injured.

Not infrequently, it was a temporary lack of this oxygen (a state called *anoxia*) or a temporary insufficiency of this oxygen (a state called *hypoxia*) that caused the original brain injury itself, regardless of the actual incident (such as a fall, a blood clot, a stoppage of breathing, a high temperature, etc.) that set in motion the chain of events that led to the undersupply of oxygen.

We did not begin this research on breathing with any idea that it might in the end be an important answer for brain-injured children. Instead, we began by looking for an answer to one of the big problems in polio and ended up with a more important answer in the treatment of brain-injured children.

Although the first love and prime interest of our little group was, and is, the brain-injured child, it was natural that in the early days we should see many patients who were not brain-injured but who had allied problems. Among them were patients suffering from polio.

It is hardly possible to express our delight at seeing the elimination of the crippler, polio. We here pay tribute to that genius, Jonas Salk, who did a better thing than merely curing those patients who had polio. He prevented polio and thus began the process of stamping it out.

One could scarcely imagine a greater pleasure, unless that pleasure were the elimination of brain injury. Here, however, there will obviously be no single answer since the problems of brain injury have a multiplicity of causes.

In the late 1940s and the early 1950s the treatment of polio was difficult work and frequently discouraging work. Polio could not be solved by treatment directed to the brain because, of course, polio was not an injury to the brain itself but instead existed along the edges of the spinal cord in what is called the anterior horn cell where nerve pathways leave the spinal cord and fan out to the various parts of the body to which they carry motor commands.

Severe polio frequently left monumental breathing problems in its wake in the form of paralyzed or partially paralyzed chest musculature. Frequently the best efforts to save the patient did not succeed, and the patient was lost in a respiratory death. All the work and effort had been to no avail.

Even when the patient did survive, there were monumental problems due to respiratory conditions. If the patient got a cold that would have been only mildly annoying to a well person, it generally resulted in pneumonia; consequently, much valuable treatment time was lost.

Furthermore, during these very frequent periods when the patient missed treatment, the progress that had been made—and it was painfully slow—was generally lost. This discouraging set of circumstances led us to the work on breathing.

What could we do to make it easier for a polio patient to combat respiratory problems? The case simply stated was this: Because of paralyzed chest musculature, the polio patient could not breathe deeply, therefore the chest capacity was bad, therefore the patient was subject to repeated respiratory attacks. It could be said that polio patients had insufficient chests.

How could we build the polio patient a "better" chest? There was already a standardized set of chest exercises to be used to increase the chest girth of well persons. However, these were dependent upon the patient's being able to carry out the exercises, something the polio patient could not do. How could one make a partially paralyzed chest (sometimes close to totally paralyzed) undertake a breathing program? If a severely involved polio patient with great respiratory problems were offered a thousand dollars for taking a very deep breath, the money would be safe because the fact was he could not. How, then, did we begin to build up a chest?

The team had in the past been faced with such a problem, the problem being: How does one make a muscle that doesn't work, work? The patient simply did not have command over the chest muscles. Faced with this problem previously in brain-injured persons, the team had come to the conclusion that, under certain circumstances, reflexes might be used to achieve motion which might be later put to volitional use by the patient. This method, called *reflex therapy,* is now in common use the world over.

Was there, then, a way in which we might have a polio patient take a deep breath by reflex activity beyond the patient's control? If we could find such a method, it was possible that we might be able to build larger chests in polio patients and eventually bring the expanded chest under the patient's command. This was the course upon which we now embarked.

Many of our efforts failed. There were those things that were partially successful but not practical. Among these was an effort to make the patient breathe reflexly by applying ice to the chest. If you simply place an ice cube against your own chest, you will realize that you take a deep breath in a reflex manner, recoiling from the cold. You will have no control over this breath; it will happen whether you want it to happen or not.

The question was, would this also happen in a polio patient? We tried it. Having bared the chest of a polio patient with a severe respiratory problem, we applied ice to his chest. The patient took a deep, deep breath, over which he himself had no control. While this method did in fact work and permitted the patient to take a deep breath without conscious control of the muscles, it did not prove to be a practical method. After three or four applications of the ice, the patient became cold and did not respond continuously to the cold application, nor was the reflex breath he took the deep rhythmic breathing that would be necessary if we hoped to improve his chest and his breathing in any reasonable period of time.

After more attempts which were unsuccessful, the group came to the realization that there was a well-known reflex for inducing deep breathing, although it had never been used in a therapeutic sense. To understand this method, you must first understand something about the way the human body regulates its oxygen supply. The human body is a most magnificent instrument and one cannot imagine a man-made machine that could match it in performance. A good example of this is the action of the chemoreceptors.

The chemoreceptors are small areas within the brain that control a complicated and vital function. These tiny chemoreceptors might be said to be a sort of laboratory, which not only gives constant laboratory reports (somewhere near twenty each minute of life) but finds and quickly solves chemical problems in the body. (At least, such problems are solved within the ability of the chemoreceptor laboratory system to do so.) The purpose of these chemoreceptors is to test every incoming breath of air. In the event that this incoming breath of air does not contain enough oxygen (or too high a level of carbon dioxide) to sustain life, the chemoreceptors not only report this fact instantaneously but *do* something about it. What the chemoreceptors do about it is to set in motion a process within the brain that, since there is not enough oxygen in the air now surrounding the human being, makes this human being breathe deeper and faster. This breathing takes place on a reflex level. As a result of this reflex breathing, the human being takes in a greater quantity of air than usual and thus is able to extract more oxygen to meet his body's needs.

We knew, therefore, that if a group of human beings sat in a room which was very tightly sealed, and thus did not get enough oxygen, as the air became more and more unpleasant and the oxygen content went down and the carbon-dioxide content went up, the people enclosed in that room would reflexly breathe faster and deeper. This is one set of circumstances that causes us to yawn in order to get more oxygen. This would compensate for the lack of oxygen as long as that were possible and therefore sustain life longer.

Now we asked ourselves: If a group of human beings, including a polio patient with a severe respiratory problem, were placed in a sealed room so that as the oxygen was used up and the oxygen content went down and the people in the room began to breathe deeper and faster reflexly, would the polio patient also breathe deeper and faster? If he would, he would be getting great chest movement even though he could not control his chest movements as could the well people. The reason we suspected this was so was that even the well people would not *consciously* be breathing deeper; they would not be breathing deeper because they ordered their chest musculature to do so, but instead because of a reflex action over which they had no control. The question then became: Was this life-saving deep-breathing reflex intact in the polio patient, as it is in well people?

Unable to answer that question in any way except by actually trying this experiment, the staff prepared such a room. The head nurse, Lorraine Bouldin, who was herself a severe polio patient with a severe respiratory problem was brought into this room along with other staff members. The room was then crudely sealed by putting paper strips under the door (it had no windows), using putty to plug up holes and then painting around the edges. Having done this, the staff sat in the room and simply breathed over a period of several hours.

Since the room was very inefficiently sealed, it was several hours before there was a significant lowering of the oxygen content, and raising of the CO_2 content, but as this occurred it was easy to see that the staff members began, on a reflex basis, to breathe deeply and rapidly. With fascinated eyes, we watched while Lorraine, in her wheel chair, also breathed more deeply and more rapidly than she was capable of doing on a volitional basis. We were elated.

However, the particular arrangements we had set up for the experiment were not such as would readily permit us to give Lorraine the treatment for (say) five minutes out of every hour, so we went to an engineer and asked him to design for us a room for the purpose. Even though the engineer offered to design such a room without charging for his services, the estimated cost turned out to be twenty-two thousand dollars. Without a special grant it was obvious we could not go this route.

As we moodily discussed this problem one evening, someone came up with a bright idea, or perhaps it would be safer to say that up to now we had been taking a very stupid approach. Why, said this staff member, is it necessary for us to have a large room? Could we not simply take a small closet, put one patient in the closet at a time, and hermetically seal the closet itself? Obviously this was a splendid idea and might reduce the cost to a point where we could afford to try the experiment.

On that happy note we began to consider how this might be done. Suddenly Colonel Anthony Flores, a top-flight U. S. Army physical educationist who had left the Army to join our team, said, "If it is true that a smaller room would not only be less expensive but better than a larger room, why do we not simply arrange a boxlike device in which the patient's upper body may be put? Why is it necessary for his lower body to be encased at all?" He had hardly finished speaking before he was interrupted by Dr. Bob, who said, "If this be so, why the upper body? Why not just the head, since it is only the breathing mechanism in which we're interested?" At which time, the speech therapist Claude Cheek quickly interrupted to say, "In fact, why not just the mouth and the nose since these are the only external breathing apparatus that are important to this question?" This was quite obviously sensible; therefore instead of a twenty-two-thousand-dollar room we substituted paper bags into which the patient might breathe.

This had actually been suggested sometime before by Fay himself

—but with a different goal in mind related to the diagnosis of certain kinds of brain injury.

The team delightedly tried this approach. We held the paper bag tightly around Lorraine's face to include the nose and the mouth; in thirty seconds the concentration of carbon dioxide in the paper bag was great enough to cause her to begin deep respiratory movements.

Claude Cheek, who had thought of the paper bag, then came to another very sensible conclusion. He suggested that the small plastic bags which had been designed for the administration of oxygen to patients might be used. These bags were inexpensive and were also disposable. This suggestion obviously had much merit since the bags were designed specifically to fit over the mouth and nose of the patient. They quickly proved to be valuable.

Now began a long period of testing. The staff, using itself as guinea pigs, set out to determine what happened, not only to respiration, but to pulse, blood pressure and so on when this bag was used. It was determined that up to a period of three minutes, at least in well persons, there were no untoward effects other than the effect of deeper, quicker respiration.

Now we began work on Lorraine herself, who, despite an overwhelming paralysis, ran the nursing staff from her wheel chair. Her respiratory problem was, in fact, a rather desperate one and she volunteered herself as a subject. She had little to lose since she was in constant danger of her life as it was. We could hardly control our elation when it became clear that this method did work and that her chest improved tremendously.

Respiratory episodes were cut way down. Her chest began to grow in size, which was startling, as Lorraine was very much an adult and therefore had been assumed to have a relatively fixed chest.

Having established, after some months, that a well person could wear the mask with some discomfort up to a period of ten minutes, and with no discomfort up to three minutes, and that no important physiological change other than the physiological effect on respiration itself took place, the team now chose, after consultation with Dr. David Reiber, the chest specialist on the staff, a period of one minute as a perfectly safe period of time to use on the patient himself.

The mask has since been used for this purpose in many institutions and many countries and is still being used today on the small remaining numbers of polio patients.

In light of the things that we have since learned, the staff now looks back with embarrassment on the period of time when the mask was used exclusively on the polio patients while the brain-injured patient whose chest breathing was as bad or worse sat side by side with the polio patient and did not receive this benefit.

It was at an evening conference a long time later that Lindley Boyer, one of the staff members who had come to us as a patient, said, "Have you ever wondered what would happen if we used the mask on the adult brain-injured patients? Do you realize how bad their posture and chest position is? In the early stages of stroke, as an example," she said, "the brain-injured patient sits slumped in his chair, therefore materially reducing his breathing. Also, because his paralyzed arm, if it is flaccid, is held in the midline or, if it is spastic, is held across his chest, there are further restrictions on his breathing. What would happen," she proposed, "if we used the breathing mask on the adult brain-injured patient?" Bob Doman spoke quickly, "How about the brain-injured children? They always have bad chests." He pointed out how frequently the brain-injured child had colds and respiratory conditions. Generally speaking, such a child had many more colds than his brothers and sisters and these lasted longer. If the colds and respiratory illnesses were accompanied by high temperatures, he frequently had convulsive seizures, as well. This was a most interesting thought, one which we felt should be approached very carefully since breathing into the mask affected the brain directly. We had more reservations about the complications that might exist here than we did in the case of polio where there was certainly no problem within the confines of the brain.

The more one thought about the idea the more intriguing it became. Certainly the brain-injured did have bad chests, frequently as bad and sometimes worse than many of the polio patients. Improving a child's chest should have good ramifications. His posture, for one thing, should be better and also he should have less respiratory episodes which would reduce his loss of treatment time. Perhaps even more important, he might be less vulnerable to the seizures that frequently followed infections of any kind in the brain-injured child.

We reviewed why it was that Temple Fay had used such breathing measures as the paper bag so long before. The fact was, we recalled from our conversations with him, he had used carbon dioxide, rebreathing, as a test. It was his feeling that, in certain types of brain injury, carbon dioxide would force relaxation and as a result of this one could do a differential diagnosis between two kinds of brain injury. He had described this in the literature and had used tests with carbon dioxide being administered by an anesthetist.

He had also told us long ago of the use of carbon dioxide in the treatment of epileptics, who were subject to seizures or convulsions. His theory had been that an epileptic undergoes a convulsion as a sort of reflex protest against a temporary insufficiency of oxygen to the brain, much as a fish out of water flops this way and that trying to get back in. Fay therefore tried administering *oxygen* during convulsive seizures. As he had stated the result, "The patients promptly had bigger and better seizures."

The experiment was a failure. However, no one knew better than Fay that carbon dioxide is one of the most powerful vasodilators known to man. This is to say, the rich content of carbon dioxide in the blood stream will cause the blood vessels to dilate or open wider thus permitting the flow of a greater *volume* of blood to the brain and, consequently, an increase in the *amount* of oxygen available to the brain. This, of course, was the reason his experiment had failed. By giving the patient oxygen he had cut *down* the carbon dioxide and thus constricted the blood vessels and as a final result *reduced* rather than *increased* oxygen to the brain.

Then, of course, Fay performed the exactly opposite experiment.

Fay now gave carbon dioxide to patients while they were having convulsive seizures. He did so with hundreds of patients. He had found that doing so had resulted in reduction in the severity of seizures, in the length of seizures and in the frequency of seizures.

It had long been recognized that the well human being operated well or badly in direct relationship to the adequacy of usable oxygen available at the brain level. If a well human being is deprived of oxygen, he can, in a five-minute cycle, go through the following stages. First, he will become inco-ordinate. Second, he will have *petit mal* seizures exactly like those minor epileptic episodes that we see so often in the brain-injured child. Next, he will become grossly inco-ordinate, be unable to walk, speech will become thick and he will drop objects held in his hands. Next, he will actually have a *grand mal* convulsive seizure, which looks exactly like those seizures that occur in a brain-injured patient. Following this, he will suffer brain damage due to the lack of oxygen to the brain cells and, last of all, he will die. This whole cycle can take place in five minutes in the well human being. It was certain that the brain-injured patient who *already* had a damaged brain needed this oxygen no less than did the well person. Therefore, if we could improve the chest capacity and breathing of the brain-injured patient, this should be of tremendous value.

Following this line of thought, we began extremely cautious experiments on the brain-injured. Having already done these experiments on the staff and having established that three minutes out of each hour was a very safe treatment level, we now began with brain-injured patients in ten-second periods. Over a period of many months, we worked up to a full minute, as we had with the polio patients.

The results were even better than we had hoped. Not only did the patient's breathing improve, but his problems with respiratory illnesses decreased. As in the case of polio patients, our brain-injured patients often had *fewer* respiratory episodes than other members of his family.

This breathing program has now been in use for many years at The Institutes as well as in many other institutions in the United States and abroad. By 1972 more than a billion maskings had been given to brain-injured children in the United States and the rest of the world.

We had found a technique that not only improved the brain's nutrition, by enriching its oxygen supply, but was sometimes even life-saving.

16.

WE PUT IT TO THE TEST

My apprenticeship to Temple Fay really stopped in 1955 when I became the director of The Institutes. Fay continued to work with us for two more years, but now I had the responsibility for forty inpatients, many critically ill, and I had to be director, administrator, chief of staff, and chief therapist. My wife, Hazel, was the head nurse, the charge nurse on each of the shifts, and sometimes the only nurse on a shift.

Having sold our house and given all of the money we possessed to The Institutes, we had inevitably moved the family into The Institutes, lock, stock and barrel. Perhaps if I said that for six months I worked twenty-four hours a day, seven days a week, and that Hazel worked longer, you would know how I felt then.

Now for the first time I could no longer give first priority to sitting at the feet of my teacher. I had patients who were counting on me.

Although all or virtually all of the theoretical constructions with which we had begun had been those of Dr. Fay, practically all of our practical applications were developed by the team working together.

Twenty years had passed since I had first met Fay and ten years had passed since I had joined with Fay. The decade of the fifties, our decade of discovery, was drawing to a close.

It seemed to us to be a time for consolidation, a time for thought, a time to decide precisely where we were going and just how we ought to get there. Four questions cried out for answering. (1) Just what *were* we? (2) What did we *believe?* (3) What were we *doing?* (4) What were the *results?*

Here's the way it looked to us in the middle of 1957.

1. Just what *were* we? We were the staff of The Rehabilitation Center at Philadelphia and we numbered about forty—physicians, therapists (physical, occupational, speech), nurses, psychologists, educators, administrators, board members, and so on.

We were a Federally tax-exempt, non-profit organization

chartered for the purpose of conducting treatment of brain-injured children and adults as well as research into all problems associated with brain injury and for teaching other professional persons what the treatment and research had revealed relative to brain function in normal and brain-injured patients.

We had forty inpatients with severe neurological disorders including twenty children and twenty adults. Fay had always been greatly excited by what he described as that "wealth of clinical material."

We had many resident students ranging from all of the senior nurses from five major Philadelphia hospitals (each of whom spent a month in residency at the Center during her senior year where she received forty hours of didactic instruction per week taught by the senior staff members) up to post-graduate students in the therapies, education or psychology to resident post-doctoral students in medicine or education from the United States and abroad.

Our research was primarily clinical, although we were soon to plunge into laboratory research as well.

Our patients were now referred to us by many physicians including Dr. Eugene Spitz, a top pediatric neurosurgeon and Dr. Edward B. LeWinn, chief of medicine at Albert Einstein Medical Center, Philadelphia, a greatly respected internist, who had earned such respect by the high order of his clinical abilities and research projects. Dr. Sigmund LeWinn, his brother, was our chief consultant in pediatrics and much liked by the staff. There were consultants in orthopedics, urology, ophthalmology and general medicine as well.

We had earned some national and even international reputation as a pioneering institution in the treatment of brain-injured patients.

2. What did we *believe?* What we believed was by now a great deal clearer than it had been. If today our beliefs sound so simple as to be obvious, I can only say that in 1957 few others found them obvious. We believed:

(a) That brain injury was in the brain. (This has always been our most radical belief.)

(b) That since the brain controls all human functions, if the brain is severely hurt the *symptoms* of brain injury will be demonstrated everywhere in the body.

(c) That treatment of the symptoms which exist in the eyes, ears, mouth, chest, arms, legs and everywhere else in the body will not alter the basic brain injury.

(d) That if we could successfully attack the problem in the brain itself rather than merely the symptoms, the symptoms would disappear spontaneously.

(e) That there were ways to address treatment to the brain itself.

Perhaps what we believed could best be summed up in a speech I had made in 1953 to Dr. Rusk's Institute for Physical Medicine and Rehabilitation. It had been something of a landmark in our progress that we had been asked to speak there because it was at that time without question the most famous rehabilitation center in the world. My lecturing fee was by far the highest I had ever received up to that time, and I had been excited and flattered at the invitation.

I said in my conclusion:

> It must then be considered as a basic principle, that when a lesion exists within the confines of the brain, that treatment, to be successful, must be directed to the brain wherein lies the cause rather than to that portion of the periphery where the symptoms are reflected. Whether the symptoms exist as an almost undetectable subtlety in human communication or in an overwhelming paralysis, this principle must not be violated by those who seek success with the brain-injured patient.

Nothing in this principle had changed by 1957. Nor has it today.

3. What were we *doing*? By 1957 a rather clear program had emerged. This program was taught to the parents by us and carried out at home under our careful supervision. We accepted as inpatients only those children who had not succeeded on a carefully conducted home program.

Whether administered by us or by the parents at home, the program was as follows:

(a) All non-walking children spent all day on the floor on their stomachs crawling (if they could) and creeping (if they could).

(b) All children were "patterned," that is to say, they would be given external help in going through the basic motions of, say, crawling if they could not yet crawl well on their own. They were patterned four times a day, five minutes each time, seven days a week, using truncal pattern (if a child could not move his limbs well), homolateral pattern (if he could not crawl well) and cross pattern (if he could not creep well). If he could walk but did it awkwardly, he was given drill in cross-pattern walking.

(c) Children who demonstrated sensory losses were given specific sensory stimulation.

(d) A program to establish clear-cut cortical hemispheric dominance was established for children who were mixed up as to which side was dominant.

(e) A masking program to improve the vital capacity of the lungs and thus give optimum oxygen to the brain was used on all children.

4. What were the *results?* By the beginning of 1958 it was clear that we were achieving results such as we had never achieved before, and it now seemed time to subject the new methods of treatment to the same kind of testing we had given the old treatment many years earlier.

This testing was made easier by the presence at The Institutes of two French research physicians. Their names were Jean and Elizabeth Zucman and they were man and wife. Dr. Jean Zucman was an orthopedic surgeon who was carrying out a one-year research program for us under the direction of Dr. Edward LeWinn, who had finally joined our staff, at first as a consultant and later as the director of the Research Institute.

Dr. Elizabeth Zucman, like my brother, Bob, was a physiatrist and was fascinated by the children's clinic which, for reasons too lengthy to describe, was held on weekends with the staff donating its time. It was to this weekend clinic that the parents who were treating their children at home returned periodically for consultation. While it may be difficult to credit, it is nonetheless true that this clinic began on Saturday morning at 8:00 A.M. and ran *without stopping* until late Sunday afternoon.

Betty Zucman, who was studying at The Institutes on a Fulbright Scholarship, worked a normal week and was not required to work those incredible weekend hours.

Still she heard rumors of some of the results being achieved with the children under our program, and although she was quite polite she obviously didn't believe them.

Would *"Monsieur Le Directeur"* permit her to attend the weekend children's clinics of which she had heard?

But of course. And so she did. She stayed awake and alert through three weekends from beginning to end. She was deeply impressed.

Would *"Monsieur Le Directeur"* permit her to attend all future clinics and might she—ah—that is—take notes?

But of course.

She took her notes. She drew her conclusions. And she chose her words carefully. The results, she reported, were not as rumored. The results were far greater than rumored. She had been skeptical to begin with, but had come away completely persuaded that something extremely important was going on.

Some severely brain-injured children were markedly improved. Despite the fact that everyone said that such was not possible, some of them were actually walking.

We *must,* she declared, carefully study the results and make a statistical evaluation of them, and we *must* do it immediately. We *must* report our findings in an article and submit that article to the most important medical journal in the United States at once. It *must* be the *Journal of the American Medical Association.* We must. We *must.* She would hear of no objections and she would hear of no delay. It *must* be done.

If it *must* be done, I had allowed, then she herself could damn well begin the statistical evaluation right now since she was a skilled medical researcher.

And so she did in a study of the children we were treating in 1958 and 1959.

The results were highly impressive compared with any other results of treatment of brain-injured children that we could find in the medical literature, and we had searched carefully. In truth, we could find no other report in the medical literature of anyone who had ever reported any positive result in the treatment of brain-injured children.

We wrote our report and argued about every word in it. We spent two whole weeks arguing about the title alone.

When we were satisfied, we submitted it to the *Journal of the A.M.A.* It was accepted, and published on September 17, 1960. That article (reprinted in its entirety as Appendix B) reported on the results achieved in the treatment of 76 severely brain-injured children, none of whom were given much chance of any significant improvement under conventional therapy. Seventy-four of the 76 made measurable progress. Twenty-one, in fact, learned to walk well and easily in full cross pattern, including 3 who had initially been unable to crawl, 6 who initially had been unable to creep, and 12 who initially had walked, but badly. Furthermore, most of the children were, at the time the study was completed, continuing to improve, having been on the program for an average of only 11 months.

Not only did the *Journal of the A.M.A.* publish the article, but they sent an advance news release to all the major newspapers and magazines in the United States telling them that a very important article about brain-injured children would appear in the next issue of the *Journal.*

We received thousands of requests for reprints and not a word of criticism about the article itself although some of the establishment thought all that newspaper publicity wasn't seemly. They wished *we* hadn't notified the newspapers.

However, it was now on record that there was new hope for an effective treatment of the brain-injured.

Clinical research is a stimulating, exhilarating, often intoxicating thing. When years of work and hope finally start paying off in terms of really producing function in severely brain-injured children, it can even be an ecstatic thing. And for us it was.

It is also a provoking, hectic, frustrating, frenetic, infuriating, demoniacal thing.

A clinic is about as far removed from the theoretical, neatly ordered, contemplative, disembodied sort of laboratory research as one can imagine.

In some kinds of pure research I suppose one can routinely stop work at five o'clock and just lock the door and go home.

But I wouldn't know. My own work has been too clinical.

One cannot lock the door at five o'clock on desperately needful children whose needs are no less desperate because they can't voice them. Face to face with a child who may be paralyzed, often gasping for breath, frequently speechless, sometimes vomiting, occasionally convulsing, and always hurt, hurt, hurt, there is little opportunity for scholarly contemplation.

We strove for order and neatness, but in the chaotic circumstances which surrounded our work, we rarely attained it.

Sometimes we worked our way tidily from theory to application. More often, we improvised, then worked back from practice to theory. Most often what ended in a new treatment began as a simple hunch, arrived at by observing a single child and checked out by observing a hundred others. A good hunch would survive scrutiny; a bad one would fall by the wayside. If the hunch was to the effect that certain kinds of children would benefit from more of A, or less of B, we'd look for ways to provide more of A or less of B. Then we'd check periodically to see whether this helped or not. That's the way it is with clinicians. It's sloppy, but you can say in its favor that it never hurts if you're careful and that it often works. In fact, this method of approaching problems accounts for most of human progress since time began.

With us there were occasions when our theory was more advanced than our practice. At other times, and more commonly, it was much the other way around, and this was certainly the case when the fifties ended.

The early years of the sixties were spent in improving methods of treatment, but with the ever-broadening group of extraordinary people who were joining us we were also coming to be able to understand much more clearly why the things we were doing worked.

There was that courageous and brilliant Brazilian surgeon, Raymundo Veras, who had brought his beloved son, José Carlos Veras, to Philadelphia for treatment and found his highly respected, dignified and orderly life torn asunder when he saw what happened to his son. He remained to become a post-graduate student when he was already in his forties. He returned to Brazil to become the founder of the Centro de Reabilitation, Nossa Senhora da Gloria, an almost exact reproduction of The Institutes in Philadelphia, and in the process of doing so his highly respected, dignified and orderly life disappeared along with his family fortune, which had been substantial. In its place came our seven-day week and twenty-hour day (which is reasonably alien to prominent families in Brazil) and a new kind of respect based not on who he was or what his name was but rather on what he did for children.

As a result of his continuing dedication, thousands of children have been helped, and another center has been established in Argentina with the help of the Aaron Maiman Foundation and under the direction of Dr. Eduardo Sequeiros.

Many other centers were soon established in South America. All have had success in treating brain-injured children paralleling the success in Philadelphia.

There was Gretchen Kerr, whom I originally didn't like and wouldn't hire. Gretchen worked for months as a volunteer before I saw my error. In a lifetime during which I had made some superb judgments about people (often against everyone's advice) and some gigantic boners about people (often against everyone's advice) my instant, instinctive, intuitive judgment that I didn't like Gretchen Kerr stands out not merely as the major mistake of my lifetime but perhaps might be the supreme misjudgment of the twentieth century. What I had seen as coldness was monumental calm. What I had seen as complete reserve was constant thoughtfulness. Today she is the director of the entire children's unit.

Three more extraordinary M.D.s had joined the permanent staff. There was Dr. Rosalise Wilkinson, a pediatrician. There was Dr. Evan Thomas, the man who had earlier done himself out of a job as one of the world's leading syphilologists by finding the answer. (After his controlled study on the effects of penicillin in the treatment of syphilis, the problem of finding an effective treatment was a problem no longer.)

They would both, in the years to come, accompany us into the most primitive countries in the world in our search for the developmental stages in children that are common to all cultures. These two, like Dr. Leland Green, internist and allergist, contributed mightily toward working out the scientific reasons why some of our methods worked as well as they did.

Two physical therapists also joined us; namely, Art Sandler and Peter Moran. Both had come because they could no longer live with themselves in the face of their failures with brain-injured children after having used classical methods of treatment.

For like reasons, Dr. Neil Harvey and Bill Wells came to us from education and human engineering respectively.

Then there was Meg Tyson, a laboratory and X-ray technician who brought us not only her specific skills but also a vast love of children, and Elaine Lee of the prodigious memory who never forgets that every folder or punched card in her files is also an individual she can call by first name.

These new staff members along with the earlier staff members and many others who have not been described threw their knowledge and weight into the battle for the kids' progress and into the understanding of that progress.

17.

SPEECH

No privilege is more important to man than the ability called speech.

Speech may be defined as the ability to assign a specific sound to symbolize an idea. In English as in most modern languages the sound is almost invariably symbolic, contrived and abstract, having no relationship to the idea except whatever relationship we assign to it. English is not an onomatopoetic language. Man agrees to visualize a specific idea when another man makes a specific sound.

In the English language we have agreed that if we hear a human being make the noise *pencil,* we will visualize a long thin object containing a lead in its core which is used to write with. There is no innate correspondence between the noise and the object. In French they have agreed that the sound *crayon* will evoke the same thought. In Portuguese they have agreed that the sound *lapis* will signify the same thing. Further sophistication of the same idea has created and refined the approach until very complicated ideas can be communicated.

In no area is man more vulnerable to misunderstanding, criticism and downright abuse from his fellow man than if he should fail to develop speech or, having gained it, should lose it—for when man loses the ability to express himself by speech he is suspect in the world of having lost, also, the senses by which he arrives at the conclusions which he would express in speech. The world feels, it might be said, that if he can't say his name, it proves that he doesn't know his name. This is as unfair as holding that if a paralyzed man doesn't walk it must necessarily be because he does not know what walking is.

The same brain injury that stops walking also frequently stops talking, as I could easily remember from my stroke cases of a dozen years earlier. Lest you, the reader, if you are young, immediately disqualify yourself from this category, let it be understood that if you are old enough to read this paragraph, you are old enough to have a stroke, for not even children are immune to this devastating problem. We have seen stroke cases at every age level from one year or less to ninety-six years of age. The child who has had a stroke resembles, tragically, in every way, the older person who has suffered a stroke.

Imagine if you can the tragic circumstances that might well occur if you yourself were to suffer a stroke—a so-called "cerebral vascular accident." The tragedy we are about to describe occurs daily all over the world and has since man first existed.

Your stroke might be caused by many circumstances. To name only two:

1. You could suffer cerebral hemorrhage; that is to say, a break in one of the arteries or capillaries or veins which carry the blood to and from the brain. This would release blood into the surrounding tissues, and could drastically interfere with the function of the affected tissues. This could happen because of an injury to the head from an automobile accident, a falling brick, a diving accident, a bullet on the battlefield, weakening brain blood vessels due to advancing age, or any number of additional reasons.

2. You could suffer a stoppage of the blood circulation to a portion of the brain, occasioned by the blocking of one of the passageways of the blood by a blood clot. This would deprive that brain tissue of its normal supply of oxygen and cause damage to that part of the brain. This could happen because you had just undergone surgery in some other part of the body, or because you (if you are female) had recently borne a child, or for a number of other reasons. Clots can form anywhere, and can move freely through the larger arteries, then clog the first smaller channel they attempt to enter.

Let us suppose that your tragedy has taken place and that at some hour of the day or night you have lost consciousness, unaware of what happened to you. After a period of unconsciousness (of which, of course, you are unaware) you might eventually waken to find yourself alone in a hospital bed. Having asked yourself where you are and why you are there, you then might attempt to get out of the bed, only to find yourself completely or partially paralyzed on the side of your body in which your handedness exists; that is to say, if you are a right handed person you might find yourself paralyzed on the right side. You might also discover that even the other side of your body did not seem to respond as well as it should, and after unsuccessful attempts to get out of bed you might lie back to ponder what has happened to you. It is not impossible that shortly thereafter a nurse might enter the room and you, much relieved, might say to the nurse, "What am I doing here, where am I, what happened to me?" But you might find, to your horror, that the words emerging from your mouth are, "Dub dub dub dub dub" or "Zuu zuu zuu zuu zuu zuu."

If the nurse then looked upset but quickly recovered to say, "Everything is fine," it would be understandable if you then said, "Everything is *not* fine, I am paralyzed and I find I am having difficulty in speaking." If what emerged from your mouth was, again, "Dub dub dub dub dub," one might well understand your distress. Let us suppose that next your family arrived. You might well try to say to your family, "Where am I and what happened to me and thank goodness you're here." If again you heard yourself say, "Dub dub dub," imagine your feelings at this time.

Let us further suppose that the family now stood at the foot of the bed and said across your totally aware body, "Isn't it terrible, he was always such a bright person." If by this time you in your frustration in attempting to make the family understand that while you can't talk you understand those things taking place about you and know very well what you want to say . . . if you pick up a bedpan and throw it at the family, this action, of course, would in no way solve the problem but would be very likely to produce this reaction, "And now not only is he off his rocker but he's becoming violent."

If this example seems impossible or overdrawn, it can only be said that, tragically, it takes place daily. We have seen many patients who, following a stroke and the loss of speech, were dealt with as if they were psychotic and eventually ended up with their bodies in restraint. In such a situation it can well be understood why the patient's anguish might quickly result in another cerebral vascular accident, perhaps the final one.

You can also well imagine the satisfaction many patients felt in their initial interview at The Institutes when the examiner, realizing instantly that the patient was *aphasic* (the proper name for the inability to communicate due to a cortical problem), said, "Mr. Jones, while you can't talk, I know perfectly well that you know what you want to say, but can't say it."

It was a great pleasure, in those days before the children crowded all the adults out of the doors of The Institutes, to watch the patient sigh a gigantic sigh of relief and say very clearly with his countenance, if not with words, "Thank the good Lord that someone knows I am not off my rocker because I can't say the things I want to say."

Perhaps the reader is saying to himself that what I have described is a terrible thing, and that while such dreadful things may have happened fifty or a hundred years ago they couldn't possibly happen today.

If you are thinking any such thing it would be prudent to disabuse yourself of the notion. It was at this time in history (the beginning of the 1960s) that a very famous man had a stroke and was paralyzed on his right side and unable to speak.

It was also at about this time in history that I was teaching a large class of professional people including physicians, therapists, psychologists and others. When I discussed this aspect of speech problems I could see disbelief on the faces of several people. This rather annoyed me.

"Very recently," I began, "a very famous man had a stroke and I understand has a speech problem. It is quite conceivable that some therapist is at this moment showing him a picture of a cat and saying, 'Ambassador, this is a *Cat*. This is the cat's *Head* and this is the cat's *Tail*.'

"This particular man," I continued, "has made a half a billion dollars. He has a son who is President of the United States, another son who is Attorney General of the United States and still another who is a Senator. I am quite confident that Joseph Kennedy knows what a cat is. Still, it is quite conceivable that he is being treated as if he were feeble-minded just because he can't talk."

Two and a half years later I had opportunity to learn that this was almost precisely what had been happening to Joseph Kennedy.

One often wonders what might happen if one day when the door opened to admit the therapist with the pictures of the cat a patient might not in sheer anguished frustration pick up an ash tray and hit the therapist right on the head. If the patient happened to hit the therapist in exactly the right spot on the head (a couple of inches above the ear, on the dominant side of the brain) with exactly the right amount of force (enough to rupture the middle cerebral artery —but not enough to kill), then there would be two people who would know what a cat was but be unable to say "cat."

While I am, in principle, pretty much opposed to anybody hitting anybody on the head, I think that in such a case I would be a good deal more in sympathy with the hitter than the hittee.

A patient who can't talk is not necessarily feeble-minded, insane or bewitched, but may simply have lost the ability to say words. What has happened to the patient is referred to in medicine as *aphasia*. Although there are many definitions of aphasia, we have chosen to define aphasia as an inability to *communicate* due to an injury in the cortex.

It is important to note that we have not used the term inability to *speak* but instead have used the term inability to *communicate*. The word *communicate* is obviously a much broader term than the term *speak*. The patient who is unable to speak due to aphasia is also unable to communicate in terms of writing, sign language, etc., and he can read only in relationship to his understanding of the spoken word. He can write only to the degree that he can talk, for aphasia is indeed a loss in the whole area of communication and not simply in the area of speech itself.

We have dealt with adults at this length because it is important to compare the problems of adult patients who have lost their powers of speech and communication with the problems of children who may never have gained speech due to brain injury. Let's return to the definition of aphasia itself, *a loss in the ability to communicate due to an injury in the cortex.* Does this description fit the children who also may not speak due to an injured cortex? It does except for one word: loss. It can't be said that a human being has lost something he didn't have in the first place. Since the children who do not speak due to a brain injury—at least those of them who incurred their injury prior to one year of age—have never spoken, it is fair to say that they cannot lose what they have never had.

In these circumstances it would obviously be improper to say that a child who had never spoken had lost his ability to speak. If this were a mere play on words it would not be important, but it is more than that. When comparing the children and the adults it is important to note that each has an advantage over the other.

The child holds over the adult one simple advantage. Let us suppose that a child was originally intended to be a right-handed child. This would mean that his left cortex would be the area responsible for his speech. Now let us suppose that prior to the time that speech had formed in that left hemisphere, the left hemisphere was hurt by brain injury. What would happen here would be a very simple thing. In the vast majority of cases, the child would simply develop speech in his *right* hemisphere instead, and this speech would be developed as well as if he had developed it in the hemisphere originally intended to carry his speech. Obviously then, in this respect the child has a tremendous advantage over the adult whose speech is firmly implanted in his left hemisphere (if he is right-handed). Only if the child is hurt in both sides of his cortex will he be truly aphasic.

What advantage does the adult have over the child? His advantage is merely this: He has known how to speak before and understands thoroughly what is required of him. The brain-injured child who may have damage in both of his hemispheres and therefore does not develop speech does not enjoy this advantage.

Let us consider now the speech problems of brain-injured children. It is certain that the majority of brain-injured children have a speech problem of one kind or another. Some of them find it difficult even to make sounds. Others can make sounds, but sounds that are without significance. Others make significant sounds but have no words. Others have a free flow of language but the voice does not have meaning. Sometimes the brain-injured child demonstrates no problem except speech.

Nothing is more vital to his wellness than the development of speech.

We had studied first the speech, or, more exactly, the lack of speech of the injured children themselves, many, many years before. We had come from that study thoroughly mystified by what we had found, or, again more precisely, what we had failed to find.

We turned next to what is called in medicine, the literature. Here, in contrast to the lack of information that had existed in relation to a well child's mobility, we found a moderate amount of information on a well child's speech and a large amount of writing on the subject of the brain-injured child's speech. However, we came away from this study even more confused than from the study of the children themselves! The things we read in this area were extremely contradictory.

This despite the fact that scientists and mothers alike had observed the development of speech carefully and recorded it carefully throughout history. There is even disagreement in the literature as to when various stages or levels of speech occur. Some observers, as an example, held that "babbling" occurred in the first month or two of life, others held that babbling began in the second year of life. Very few, if any, had defined babbling. When one turned to the dictionary he found babbling defined as babylike talking, the talking of an idiot, or the sound made by a brook.

Some of the disagreement as to when things occurred was unquestionably due to the fact that the language describing language was highly inexact, and babbling or cooing obviously meant different things to different observers.

Also, as has been noted, much of what had been recorded about the speech of well children appeared to us to be true but not significant. The word *significant* in scientific usage does not mean exactly the same thing as in normal usage. Perhaps this can best be explained with an obvious example of a true but not significant observation.

Suppose one studied a thousand children under one year old and noted that the vast majority of them did not have speech. Suppose one then studied a thousand twenty-year-olds and noted that a thousand of them did have speech. He might then properly observe that those people who have speech are a great deal taller than those people who did not have speech, and while this would be true he would have to be careful not to come to the conclusion that speech was a result of getting taller.

It was our opinion that while babbling, cooing and various other babylike sounds occurred along the way in the development of speech, these did not have to be present in themselves for the creation of speech but were merely a method of measuring the development of that speech rather than the reasons for the development of that speech. So again we returned to the well children themselves, and were now not surprised at all to find that there were again four significant stages in the development of speech in a child and that these four stages again paralleled in chronological span and in development the four stages which we had now seen many times.

These four stages are:

Stage one. The child actually begins life itself with a birth cry, which is reflex in nature and has its developmental utility but is not significant in terms of communication. This cry of the infant denotes nothing more than the presence of life itself, and when mother hears the cry she learns nothing except that the child is alive. This cry carries no message of happiness or unhappiness. The factor to measure at this level is the mere presence or absence of the ability to cry or make other sounds.

Stage two. The infant can now convey by sound the fact that he is experiencing severe pain which may actually threaten his existence and these sounds are, in essence, a cry for help. Mother recognizes quickly the imperativeness of this cry, day or night, and responds to it immediately and instinctively.

Stage three. This is the stage of significant, meaningful sound, short of language but beyond the simple cry for help. In this stage the child can convey pleasure, displeasure, apprehension, anticipation and other states of happiness or unhappiness. The world recognizes cooing, for instance, as indicating happiness. The significance of this stage lies not so much in the newfound ability to make varying sounds by varying mouth positions and breath control but is instead in the fact that each variation is now meaningful and conveys a clear, although limited, message. The factor to measure here is whether or not these sounds are meaningful to mother even though no words yet exist. This stage is goal-directed, and the child can get many things he wants although he has no words.

Stage four. At this level the baby actually begins to imitate the sounds he hears and to use them meaningfully. It matters not to the central nervous system whether these words happen to be English, French, Portuguese or whatever. It is significant only that the nervous system has matured to the point where it can now deal in symbolic sounds. The baby begins to say single words and to establish a vocabulary. His language will continue to improve in scope and meaning until around six years of life at which time the significant brain maturation will be complete. This obviously does not mean that his ability to improve in speech stops at six, but the difference between a laconic adult and an adult with the eloquence of Winston Churchill is not dependent upon simple maturation but rather upon many, many factors which space will not permit us to touch upon.

Now that we felt that we understood the basic stages of speech growth, the next question was: What can we do about the speech problems of the brain-injured child?

We had not been impressed with the results of speech therapy in the brain-injured children. Indeed we did not believe we had ever seen a child speechless due to a brain injury who had learned to speak as a result of the standard methods of speech therapy.

Our belief, which was now very strong, that when an injury existed in the brain, it was the brain you had to treat, seemed to hold true in the case of the absence of speech. We concluded that a child could not have his speech problem solved by dealing with his tongue, mouth, lips and larynx any more than a child could have his walking problems solved by dealing with his feet, knees, ankles or hips, if the reason for both of these problems existed within the brain. We were then totally unaware that as our new treatment methods progressed we had been developing adequate methods of training the brain-injured child to talk, by treating his brain and then simply giving him opportunity to talk.

18.

READING

The parent of a severely brain-injured child who comes to this chapter entitled *Reading* may well be astonished at the thought that a brain-injured child with a problem in talking might be far enough along to have a problem in reading.

The mere fact that such a chapter exists in a book on brain-injured children delights us, and we cannot help but reminisce about the pathway that led us so far in a mere decade or so of time.

Just a decade or so ago it had been our goal to make the child with a severe brain-injury move just a little. Later it was our goal to make the child move just a little more. When we had succeeded in doing this with some regularity, it then became our goal to make the child walk. When we began to accomplish this in many children, it became our goal to make him walk normally.

Once it was our limited goal to help the child with a severe brain injury to make meaningful, if limited, sounds. Then it became our goal to make him speak just a little more. And then it was our goal to make him speak normally.

When this had sometimes been accomplished, it became our goal to get the child into a school, any school. Still later, it was our goal to get the child into a school with well children, no matter how far behind he might be. Still later, it was our goal to get him into a school with well children of the proper age, even though he was at the bottom of his class. Finally it became our goal to have him keep up with his peers in every way, in school and out. Let me make haste to point out that we do not mean to imply that this is always *possible* but at least today it is *always* our goal.

I should like to hazard a guess that many of you who are parents of brain-injured children are saying at this point, "I should be so happy if our child could only walk or talk and never mind being able to read."

I cannot help but remember an incident that took place a long,

long time ago when I had just finished my schooling and had taken my place as a staff member of a large hospital. I remember very clearly the attractive thirty-year-old woman who was diagnosed as having an incurable illness. This illness not only prevented walking and most other movements but was quite painful since her legs frequently flexed involuntarily, pulling up on her chest and causing great pain.

I remember well the patient's tearful request which began with the explanation that she understood she could never possibly walk, but, she said, "If only the terrible pain would stop." This patient was treated long and arduously and the day did come when the pain stopped. The patient then said, "I know I shall never be able to move, but if only I could wiggle my feet a little bit it would feel so good to know they were mine." And after much work and effort some leg movement was achieved. The patient then said that she knew she could never function or perform, but if only, using her arms, she could put a little weight on her feet, how good it would be to feel herself in the upright position. After more months of work this was accomplished. This time the patient said she knew she could never walk, but if only she could lift one foot and the other as she stood supporting herself with her arms . . . and this too was accomplished. And by this time it began to appear as if indeed the miracle of walking itself was possible. I will not soon forget the day when she was to take her first steps. It was a dramatic moment. Many of the principal members of the hospital staff were present that day in the exercise department when the patient was stood up and told to take her first steps. She walked across an entire room unsupported, and I remember waiting anxiously for the first words she would say after this miraculous accomplishment because I was sure they would be words to cherish forever. It is true that what she said was not soon to be forgotten. Having walked across the room, she turned to the delighted staff and snarled, "Does this mean I'm going to limp?"

Her miraculous recovery was a remarkable example of great good fortune and very bad diagnosis. Each time we hear a parent say, "I would be so pleased if only my child could get to do this, that or the other thing," I am reminded of that patient so long ago.

The fact is that today brain-injured children only two and three years old regularly learn to read on The Institutes' program. It was Tommy Lunski who opened our eyes. It was difficult for us to believe the absurd story that Mr. Lunski told us about Tommy. And this is strange, because when we first saw Tommy at The Institutes we were already aware of all the things we needed to know in order to understand what was happening to Tommy.

Tommy was the fourth child in the Lunski family. The Lunski parents hadn't had much time for formal schooling and had worked very hard to support their three nice, normal children. By the time Tommy was born Mr. Lunski owned a taproom and things were looking up.

However, Tommy was born very severely brain-injured. When he was two years old he was admitted for neurosurgical examination at a fine hospital in New Jersey. The day Tommy was discharged the chief neurosurgeon had a frank talk with Mr. and Mrs. Lunski. The doctor explained that his studies had shown that Tommy was a vegetablelike child who would never walk or talk and should therefore be placed in an institution for life.

All of Mr. Lunski's determined Polish ancestry reinforced his American stubbornness as he stood up to his great height, hitched up his considerable girth and announced, "Doc, you're all mixed up. That's *our* kid."

The Lunskis spent many months searching for someone who would tell them that it didn't necessarily have to be that way. The answers were all the same.

By Tommy's third birthday, however, they had found a competent neurosurgeon.

After carefully making his own neurosurgical studies, he told the parents that while Tommy was indeed severely brain-injured, perhaps something might be done for him at a group of institutions in a suburb of Philadelphia called Chestnut Hill.

Tommy arrived at The Institutes for the Achievement of Human Potential when he was just three years and two weeks old. He could not move or talk.

Tommy's brain injury and his resultant problems were evaluated at The Institutes. A treatment program was prescribed for Tommy. The parents were taught how to carry out this program at home and were told that if they adhered to it without failure, Tommy might be greatly improved.

There was no question but that the Lunskis would follow the strict program. They did so with religious intensity.

By the time they returned for the second visit, Tommy could crawl.

Now the Lunskis attacked the program with energy inspired by success. So determined were they that when their car broke down on the way to Philadelphia for the third visit, they simply bought a used car and continued to their appointment. They could hardly wait to tell us that Tommy could now say his first two words—"Mommy" and "Daddy." Tommy was now three and a half and could creep on hands and knees. Then his mother tried something only a mother would try with a child like Tommy. In much the same manner that a father buys a football for his infant son, Mother bought an alphabet book for her three-and-a-half-year-old, severely brain-injured, two-word-speaking son. Tommy, she announced, was very bright, whether he could walk and talk or not. Anyone who had any sense could see it simply by looking in his eyes!

While our tests for intelligence in brain-injured children during those days were a good deal more involved than Mrs. Lunski's, they were no more accurate than hers. We agreed that Tommy was intelligent all right, but to teach a brain-injured three-and-a-half-year-old to read—well, that was another question.

We therefore paid very little attention when Mrs. Lunski later announced that Tommy, then four years of age, could read *all* of the *words* in the alphabet book even more easily than he could read the letters. We were more concerned and pleased with his speech, which was progressing constantly, as was his physical mobility.

By the time Tommy was four years and two months old his father announced that he could read all of a Dr. Seuss book called *Green Eggs and Ham*. We smiled politely and noted how remarkably Tommy's speech and movement were improving.

When Tommy was four years and six months old Mr. Lunski announced that Tommy could read, and had read, *all* of the Dr. Seuss books. We noted on the chart that Tommy was progressing beautifully, as well as the fact that Mr. Lunski "said" Tommy could read.

When Tommy arrived for his eleventh visit he had just had his fifth birthday. Although we were delighted with the superb advances Tommy was making, there was nothing to indicate at the beginning of the visit that this day would be an important one for all children. Nothing, that is, except Mr. Lunski's usual nonsensical report. Tommy, Mr. Lunski announced, could now read anything, including the *Reader's Digest,* and what was more, he could understand it, and what was more than that, he'd started doing it before his fifth birthday.

We were saved from the necessity of having to comment on this by the arrival of one of the kitchen staff with our lunch—tomato juice and a hamburger. Mr. Lunski, noting our lack of response, took a piece of paper from the desk and wrote, "Glenn Doman likes to drink tomato juice and eat hamburger."

Tommy, following his father's instructions, read this easily and with the proper accents and inflections. He did not hesitate as does the seven-year-old, reading each word separately without understanding of the sentence itself.

"Write another sentence," we said slowly. Mr. Lunski wrote, "Tommy's daddy likes to drink beer and whiskey. He has a great big fat belly from drinking beer and whiskey at Tommy's Tavern."

Tommy had read only the first three words aloud when he began to laugh. The funny part about Dad's belly was down on the fourth line since Mr. Lunski was writing in large letters.

This severely brain-injured little child was actually reading much faster than he was reciting the words aloud at his normal speaking rate. Tommy was not only reading, he was speed-reading, and his comprehension was obvious!

The fact that we were thunderstruck was written on our faces. We turned to Mr. Lunski.

"I've been telling you he can read," said Mr. Lunski.

After that day none of us would ever be the same, for this was the last piece of puzzle in a pattern that had been forming for more than twenty years.

Tommy had taught us that even a severely brain-injured child can learn to read far earlier than normal children usually do.

Tommy, of course, was immediately subjected to full-scale testing by a group of experts who were brought from Washington for this purpose within a week. Tommy—severely brain-injured and just barely five years old—could read better than the average child twice his age—and with complete comprehension.

By the time Tommy was six he walked, although this was relatively new to him and he was still a little shaky; he read at the sixth-grade level (eleven-to-twelve-year-old level). Tommy was not going to spend his life in an institution, but his parents were looking for a "special" school to put Tommy in come the following September. Special *high,* that is, not special low. Fortunately there are a few experimental schools now for exceptional "gifted" children. Tommy has had the dubious "gift" of severe brain injury and the unquestionable gift of parents who love him very much indeed and who believed that at least one kid wasn't achieving his potential.

Tommy, in the end, was a catalyst for twenty years of study. Maybe it would be more accurate to say he was a fuse for an explosive charge that had been growing in force for twenty years.

The fascinating thing was that Tommy *wanted* very much to read and enjoyed it tremendously.

A revolution was already underway, and the cause of the revolution was television.

The kids didn't know that they would be able to read if the tools were given them, and the adults in the television industry, who finally furnished them, knew neither that the children had the ability nor that television would supply the tools that would bring about the gentle revolution.

It's astonishing really, that the secret has not been discovered by more kids long before this. It's a wonder that they, with all their brightness—because bright they are—didn't catch on.

The only reason some adult hasn't given the secret away to the two-year-olds is that we adults haven't known it either. Of course, if we had known, we would never have allowed it to remain a secret because it's far too important to the kids and to us too.

The trouble is that we have made the print too small.

The trouble is that we have made the print too small.

The trouble is that we have made the print too small.

The trouble is that we have made the print too small.

It is even possible to make the print too small for an adult's sophisticated visual pathway—which includes the brain.

It is almost impossible to make the print too big to read.

But it *is* possible to make it too small, and that's just what we've done.

We have tended to keep type so small that the typical child of preschool age simply fails to notice that words differ one from another. He can see, all right. As any mother knows, he has no trouble "seeing" a pin lying on the floor, or an ant crawling on the ground. He may not, however, have "noticed" that words differ, just as many an adult has never troubled to take notice of the difference between a bee and a wasp.

The secret is simply to make it easy for him to notice that printed words do differ. And television has now given away the secret—through the commercials.

When the man on television says, "Gulf, Gulf, Gulf," in a nice, clear, loud voice and the television screen shows the word GULF in nice, clear, big letters, the kids all learn to recognize the word—and they don't even know the alphabet.

For the truth is that very young children can read, provided that, in the beginning, you make the print very big.

But isn't it easier for a child to understand a spoken word rather than a written one? Not at all. The child's brain, which is the only organ that has learning capacity, "hears" the clear, loud television words through the ear and interprets them as only the brain can. Simultaneously, the child's brain "sees" the big, clear television words through his eye and interprets them in exactly the same manner.

It makes no difference to the brain whether it "sees" a sight or "hears" a sound. It can understand both equally well. All that is required is that the sounds be loud enough and clear enough for the ear to hear and the words big enough and clear enough for the eye to see so that the brain can interpret them—the former we have done but the latter we have failed to do.

People have probably always talked to children in a louder voice than they use with adults, and we still do so, instinctively realizing that children cannot hear and simultaneously understand normal adult conversational tones.

Nobody would think of talking to one-year-olds in a normal voice —we all virtually shout at them.

Try talking to a two-year-old in a conversational tone and chances are that he will neither hear nor understand you. It is likely that if his back is turned he will not even pay attention to you.

Even a three-year-old, if spoken to in a conversational tone, is unlikely to understand or even heed you if there are conflicting sounds or another conversation in the room.

Everyone talks loudly to children, and the younger the child is the louder we talk.

Suppose, for the sake of argument, that we adults had long ago decided to speak to each other in sounds just soft enough so that no child could hear and understand them. Suppose, however, that these sounds were just loud enough for his auditory pathway to have become sufficiently sophisticated to hear and understand soft sounds when he got to be six years of age.

Under this set of circumstances we would probably give children "hearing readiness" tests at six years of age. If we found that he could "hear" but not understand words (which would certainly be the case, since his auditory pathway could not distinguish soft sounds until now), it is possible that we would now introduce him to the spoken language by saying the letter A to him, and then B, and so on until he had learned the alphabet, before beginning to teach him how words sound.

One is led to conclude that perhaps there would be a great many children with a problem of "hearing" words and sentences, and perhaps a popular book called *Why Johnny Can't Hear*.

The above is precisely what we have done with written language. We have made it too small for the child to "see and understand."

Now let's make another supposition.

If we had spoken in whispers while simultaneously writing words and sentences very large and distinct, very young children would be able to read but would be unable to understand verbal language.

Now suppose that television were introduced with its big written words and accompanying loud spoken words. Naturally all kids could read the words, but there would also be many children who would begin to understand the spoken word at the astonishing age of two or three.

And that, in reverse, is what is happening today in reading!

TV has also shown us several other interesting things about children.

The first is that youngsters watch most "kiddie programs" without paying constant attention; but as everyone knows, when the commercials come on the children run to the television set to *hear* about and *read* about what the products contain and what they are supposed to do.

The point here is not that television commercials are pitched to the two-year-old set, nor is it that gasoline or what it contains has any special fascination for two-year-olds, because it does not. The truth is that the children can *learn* from commercials with the big enough, clear enough, loud enough, repeated message and that all children have a rage to learn.

Children would rather *learn* about something than simply be amused by a Happy Harry—and that's a fact.

As a result then, the kids ride down the road in the family car and blithely read the Esso sign, the Gulf sign and the Coca-Cola sign as well as many others—and that's a fact.

There is no need to ask the question, *"Can* very small children learn to read?" They've answered that, they *can*.

I have already described the method by which children on The Institutes' program learn to read in my book *How to Teach Your Baby to Read* (Random House, 1964).

1960 to 1970
THE DECADE OF EXPANSION

Ferris Alger
J. Michael Armentrout
Sandra Brown
Walter Burke
Frank Cliffe
Patrick Coyne
Raymond Dart, M.D.
Janet Doman
Maria Drea
Connie Ellopoulos
Fred Erdtmann
Mr. and Mrs. Rogers Follansbee
Dave Garroway
Margaret George (Canada)
Leland Green, M.D.
Harry Guenther
Neil Harvey, Ph.D.
Gretchen Kerr
Elaine Lee
Pearl LeWinn
Rosalie Gabriel
William MacNutt

Mr. and Mrs. William McMillan
Robert Morris
Peter Moran
Nathan Rachmel
Richard Ransom
Harriet Richman, Selma O'Hara,
 Claire Gold, and all the *Friends*
 of The Institutes
Cathy Ruhling
Arthur Sandler
Eduardo Sequeiros, M.D.
 (Argentina)
Vicki Thornber
Evan Thomas, M.D.
Meg Tyson
Lloyd Wells
William Wells
Roselise Wilkinson, M.D.
Dr. and Mrs. Tohru Higashi
Mr. and Mrs. Robert Magee
Bertha White
Jacqueline Schweighauser

THE INSTITUTES'
DEVELOPMENTAL
PROFILE

BRAIN STAGE		TIME FRAME		VISUAL COMPETENCE	AUDITORY COMPETENCE	TACTILE COMPETENCE
VII	SOPHISTI- CATED CORTEX	Superior Average Slow	36 Mon. 72 Mon. 108 Mon.	Reading words using a dominant eye consistent with the dominant hemisphere	Understanding of complete vocabulary and proper sentences with proper ear	Tactile identification of objects using a hand consistent with hemispheric dominance
VI	PRIMITIVE CORTEX	Superior Average Slow	22 Mon. 36 Mon. 70 Mon.	Identification of visual symbols and letters within experience	Understanding of 2000 words and simple sentences	Description of objects by tactile means
V	EARLY CORTEX	Superior Average Slow	13 Mon. 18 Mon. 36 Mon.	Differentiation of similar but unlike simple visual symbols	Understanding of 10 to 25 words and two word couplets	Tactile differentiation of similar but unlike objects
IV	INITIAL CORTEX	Superior Average Slow	8 Mon. 12 Mon. 22 Mon.	Convergence of vision resulting in simple depth perception	Understanding of two words of speech	Tactile understanding of the third dimension in objects which appear to be flat
III	MIDBRAIN	Superior Average Slow	4 Mon. 7 Mon. 12 Mon.	Appreciation of detail within a configuration	Appreciation of meaningful sounds	Appreciation of gnostic sensation
II	PONS	Superior Average Slow	1 Mon. 2.5 Mon. 4 Mon.	Outline perception	Vital response to threatening sounds	Perception of vital sensation
I	MEDULLA and CORD	Superior Average Slow	Birth to .5 Birth to 1.0 Birth to 1.5	Light reflex	Startle reflex	Babinski reflex

THE INSTITUTES DEVELOPMENTAL PROFILE

BY GLENN J. DOMAN,

	MOBILITY	LANGUAGE	MANUAL COMPETENCE
	Using a leg in a skilled role which is consistent with the dominant hemisphere	Complete vocabulary and proper sentence structure	Using a hand to write which is consistent with the dominant hemisphere
	Walking and running in complete cross pattern	2000 words of language and short sentences	Bimanual function with one hand in a dominant role
	Walking with arms freed from the primary balance role	10 to 25 words of language and two word couplets	Cortical opposition bilaterally and simultaneously
	Walking with arms used in a primary balance role most frequently at or above shoulder height	Two words of speech used spontaneously and meaningfully	Cortical opposition in either hand
	Creeping on hands and knees, culminating in cross pattern creeping	Creation of meaningful sounds	Prehensile grasp
	Crawling in the prone position culminating in cross pattern crawling	Vital crying in response to threats to life	Vital release
	Movement of arms and legs without bodily movement	Birth cry and crying	Grasp reflex

THE INSTITUTES FOR
THE ACHIEVEMENT OF
HUMAN POTENTIAL
8801 STENTON AVENUE
PHILADELPHIA, PA. 19118

NEUROLOGICAL
ORGANIZATION

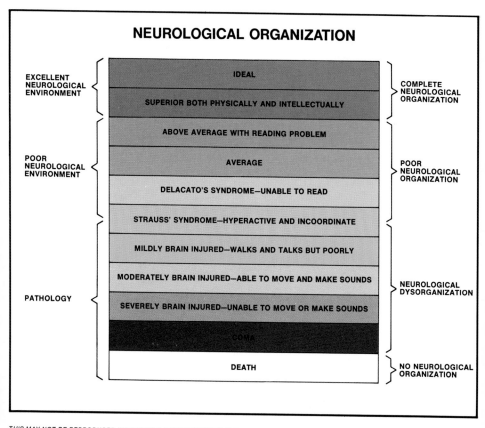

NEUROLOGICAL ORGANIZATION

EXCELLENT NEUROLOGICAL ENVIRONMENT

POOR NEUROLOGICAL ENVIRONMENT

PATHOLOGY

IDEAL

SUPERIOR BOTH PHYSICALLY AND INTELLECTUALLY

ABOVE AVERAGE WITH READING PROBLEM

AVERAGE

DELACATO'S SYNDROME—UNABLE TO READ

STRAUSS' SYNDROME—HYPERACTIVE AND INCOORDINATE

MILDLY BRAIN INJURED—WALKS AND TALKS BUT POORLY

MODERATELY BRAIN INJURED—ABLE TO MOVE AND MAKE SOUNDS

SEVERELY BRAIN INJURED—UNABLE TO MOVE OR MAKE SOUNDS

COMA

DEATH

COMPLETE NEUROLOGICAL ORGANIZATION

POOR NEUROLOGICAL ORGANIZATION

NEUROLOGICAL DYSORGANIZATION

NO NEUROLOGICAL ORGANIZATION

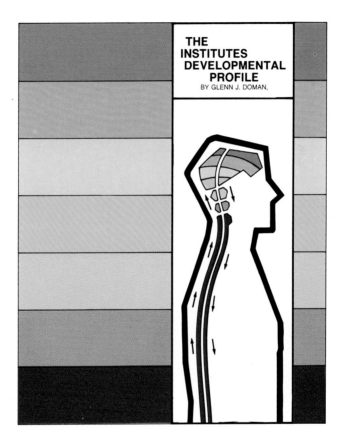

**THE
INSTITUTES
DEVELOPMENTAL
PROFILE**
BY GLENN J. DOMAN,

19.

FINDING THE BREAK
IN THE CIRCUIT

As the decade of the nineteen-sixties began a couple of related facts emerged.

First: While brain-injured children had a great deal in common, it was obvious that no two brain injuries were precisely alike. It was equally obvious that the differences between the children were a direct reflection of the differences between the location and the degree of their brain injuries. It was obvious that if we could determine in a more precise way exactly what a child could not do of the things he *should* do, we could then prescribe a program tailored *exactly* to his needs.

Second: We had by now measured literally thousands of children (including many hundreds who appeared to be totally well) to find out precisely what they could do. Somewhere within that vast amount of data there had to be a pattern, a vitally important pattern.

For at least five years I had had stronger and stronger feelings that deep within me I already *knew* that pattern and that if I just sat and thought and thought and thought I would be able to pull that pattern from my knowledge.

There were certain things that I already knew.

I knew that there were six different, important, measurable functions, the lack of which indicated trouble within the cortex. Three of these were expressive (motor) skills; namely, walking, speaking and certain manual skills culminating in writing. Three were receptive (sensory) skills; namely, reading, understanding speech and identifying objects by feel. On the road to mastery of each of these six skills, every individual went through four or more predictable stages.

I knew that what we were searching for was a pattern of growth, the grand plan, the design of how a human being got to be a human being.

It was the developmental schema we were looking for. Not *my* developmental schema, not *our* developmental schema, but nature's schema.

I knew that this was a schema of brain growth rather than physical growth.

I knew that the process ended far before physical maturity and probably before ten years of age.

I even had a name for it (which I had mentioned to no one.) I called it the *developmental profile.* It was a profile of how a child's brain matured.

I was confident that we had every piece of the puzzle within our grasp and had had for some time. The question was, which of hundreds of thousands of pieces of information were the truly significant ones? Which really mattered? Which were rungs in the ladder and which were effects rather than causes? We had a pretty clear idea of that up to one year old—but not beyond.

It was like having a song right on the edge of my mind to which I couldn't remember either the words or the music. It was maddening. Never entirely out of mind. Most of the time on the edge of my mind. Sometimes occupying most of my mind but occasionally driving everything else from it. But instead of going on for hours it had been going on for years. I had to bring that picture of a normal child into focus.

Then one of the head nurses, Florence Sharp, said something that made things start to fall in place. She was primarily responsible for the inpatient children, and that morning I asked her a question about a specific child (that same question that was driving me mad about all the children).

"How," I had asked, "is Mark doing?"

Sharpie said, "He is *much, much* better."

"Sharpie," I said irritably (and unreasonably), "how much better is *much, much* better? And don't tell me that *much, much better* is better than *much better* but not as good as *much, much, much better.*" I don't really know why I should have given Sharpie a bad time for not knowing the answer to a question that had been driving me mad for years.

"He is better."

It made me want to scream.

If he is better, then everything is peachy keen. But is it?

I had watched kids go down the drain because they were *not* better for twenty years, but I had also watched some kids go down the drain because they *were* better. Remember the kids we had found who were *better* in our original study? More than a third of them were *better*. Remember that Johnny could hold his head up better and that Mary was less spastic. But remember too, that if they had continued to get *better* at the same rate, it would have taken them until they were a hundred years old to begin to walk.

Every time I thought of this dilemma I thought of a close friend of mine and the response he always gave when anyone asked him, "How's your wife?" He would counter with a grave expression on his face and a twinkle in his eye, "Compared to whom?"

That was the heart of the question about the brain-injured child who was *better*. Better compared to whom?

Historically, that question had always been answered by comparing him to himself, which is to say by comparing him to a brain-injured child.

If an automobile that had been smashed in an accident were always compared to an automobile smashed in an accident instead of to an undamaged car, how in the world would you ever hope to fix it?

Thus, if a brain-injured child were compared only with himself and were even a tiny fraction better we might be satisfied—and that satisfaction would destroy him.

And what tools had we used to make even *that* distinction? There were two kinds of tests, but they were equally irrelevant when applied to brain-injured children.

First, there were the physical tests. These were muscle tests in which each of the hundreds of muscles in the body were individually tested by the therapist who assigned a score to each. The score might range from 0 to 10 with 0 representing total paralysis and 10 representing total strength.

In brain-injured children these tests were totally unreliable (which is to say, that five different therapists might give five different scores when testing the same muscle).

In addition, there was no sensible way to add up the results. As an example, if one tested a hundred muscles he ended up with a hundred scores. Did he, then, add them up and divide by 100 to get an average score? Let's suppose that half of the muscles tested at 0 and half tested at 10. That would give us a total of 0 and 500 to add together to come up with a total of 500. If we now divided by 100 to get an average, we would come up with an average of 5. Thus, a child who had half of his muscles totally paralyzed and half of his muscles at full strength would come up with a score of 5, showing that he was precisely in the middle, which would represent a total untruth and would describe no single muscle in his body. If, on the other hand, we regarded each of the hundred muscles individually and on a subsequent visit found thirty of his muscles to be improved by 1 point each and thirty of his muscles to have weakened by 1 point, the question would remain, was he better or worse than at the previous visit, and compared to whom?

Finally, there was the fact that the tests were not valid for the simple reason that we were testing the wrong thing. We were not testing his brain function, we were testing his biceps strength.

Testing his intelligence was even harder than testing his muscles.

The tests that are commonly used to test intelligence in the United States such as the Stanford-Binet and the Wechsler Bellevue or WISC are *reasonably* reliable and *reasonably* valid tests of a well child's *abilities*. They are nothing more. There is a great and growing suspicion on the part of almost everyone who uses them that they do not in fact test true intelligence *even* in the well child.

When these tests are used on brain-injured children they are an almost precise test of his *disabilities*. Now there is nothing wrong with testing abilities, and there is certainly nothing wrong with testing *disabilities*. Providing one gigantic proviso: Providing that when we are testing abilities we *know* we are testing abilities, and providing that when we are testing *disabilities* we *know* we are testing disabilities. But when we test disability and believe we are testing ability, only devastating results can follow, and that is precisely what occurs every single time we apply such tests to a brain-injured child. Yet the tests continue to be given and, worse, the ratings that result are often accepted as a basis for action. Brain-injured children by the hundreds of thousands have been "put away" in institutions for life on such evidence.

We knew this and knew it to be a tragedy. It was not enough, however, to know that these tests should not be relied upon in evaluating brain-injured children. We needed to come up with an acceptable alternative.

It was painfully clear why these so-called intelligence tests did not work. Every one of them depended on one or more of three possibilities.

If a child was over six, he was expected to take a test involving reading the questions and writing answers. If, because he was brain-injured, he was unable to read or write, it would be assumed that he had failed the test because he was not intelligent enough to read and write. That would get him the score of a total idiot if he was totally unable to read or write due to his brain injury or that of a moron or imbecile if he could read or write only a little due to his brain injury.

If a child was under six, or if it was recognized that the reason he couldn't read or write was due to brain injury and not to idiocy, he would be given a verbal test. The examiner would ask verbal questions and expect verbal answers. Now if he was unable to speak, due to brain injury, he would be rated an idiot on the assumption that he was not "intelligent" enough to answer the question. If he could, as a result of a lesser brain injury, answer only partially, due to the speech problem, he would come up with a score of imbecile or moron.

If a child was under three, or if it was recognized that the reason he was unable to carry on a conversation was because he was brain-injured rather than because he was an idiot, then he would be given a test that did not require him to answer the questions but simply to follow directions such as "go close the door." Now if a child was paralyzed due to brain injury and thus was unable to "go close the door," then it would be assumed that he was an idiot because he was not "intelligent" enough to go close the door.

If a very bright and sensitive examiner recognized that the reason he did not close the door was because he was paralyzed and not because he was too stupid, the examiner might fall into the final trap. He might take some function he had seen the child perform and therefore knew that the child could do, let's say rubbing his eyes; he might ask the child to do that to see if he was bright enough to understand the question. Now if the child had an auditory problem due to his brain injury and as a result was unable to interpret the question, even our sensitive examiner might well conclude that he was a complete idiot.

It happens all the time.

I am appalled that in this nation which prides itself on the fact that even a confessed murderer has many courts of appeal before he can be institutionalized for life, a child whose greatest sin is that he is hurt can be institutionalized for life—and in an institution which is almost invariably far worse than any criminal would put up with.

But that's all today and my conversation with Sharpie was back in 1960 and things were even worse then. In those days we knew with horrible certainty what was wrong with measurement. But we didn't know what was right.

The tangle began to unwind for me when Sharpie answered my question. Despite the unreasonable way in which I had asked it, Sharpie answered me softly and with understanding of my frustration.

"What I mean by *much, much better,*" she said, "is that when we saw him first a year ago he was four years old but he was behaving like a well six-month-old. Now he is five years old and behaving like a well two-year-old."

"Sharpie, that's about the first sensible thing I've heard anybody say about how a kid's doing."

"Ummmm," she said and smiled. "You always say you want sense from the staff."

"That just might be brilliant, Sharpie."

"You mean I said something brilliant?" asked Sharpie.

"Ummmm," I said and smiled.

I headed north on campus from Clarke Hall where I'd been talking to Sharpie toward the Blackburn Building where we lived. I stopped for a while on a bench in a sun that was warm for March.

I had the feeling once again that I was right on the edge of under-standing, and I thought very slowly so as not to lose my place.

If Mark had been four years old acting like a six-month-old, it meant that until we saw him first it had taken him forty-eight months to grow six months' worth, so his total progress had only been ⅛ of what it should have been.

Now if in the year that we had been seeing him he had gained a year in age but a year and a half in performance that was obviously great! His rate of progress had jumped from ⅛ of normal to 1½ times normal.

Normal? What was normal? Was it—could it be—as simple as say-ing that a five-year-old is normal when he can do what other well five-year-olds can do when they are five years old?

Now my mind was racing and all attempts to make it move slowly went out the window. I literally ran to my house. I ran into the house and to my den and locked the door. I gathered pencils, pen, papers, colored crayons, thumbtacks.

I switched on the light over my drawing board and tacked down a large piece of drawing paper.

At the top I printed

"THE DEVELOPMENTAL PROFILE"

I didn't print it very well. I was out of breath from running and highly excited and my hand shook.

If I could do what I was beginning to believe I could do, I would have a simple, workable, valid, reliable and relevant tool for meas-uring the degree of disability and rate of progress of brain-injured kids. Without the ability to measure there can be no science, and I had been disturbed by our lack of ability to measure our own results for many years. If it worked, we could *measure* our results—both our successes and our failures. It was impossible to say which was the most important.

Good-by, thank God, to expressions such as "he looks better," which I had listened to in treatment facilities around the world for years. Indeed, any statement to the effect that a child "looks better" had long since been banned at The Institutes. (If somebody slipped and said it, there was a standard answer: "Don't tell me he looks better. I'm not interested in your lousy opinion. What can he *do* that he *couldn't* do before?")

No wonder I had long felt on the edge of it. For years we had been asking each other, "What can he do that he couldn't do before?" That was the key.

Now I believed that might be the key to Nature's grand design. So simple. So clear. It had always been there, right before my eyes.

No wonder I couldn't find it. The obvious is always the most difficult to appreciate.

I got to work.

How had Sharpie known that Mark had been behaving like a six-month-old a year ago?

That was simple. We had measured hundreds of well six-month-olds. A well six-month-old could crawl but not creep. He could make some meaningful sounds but not all of them. He had a grasp reflex and he could let go. He had pretty good vision and could see outlines very well. He could understand a good many meaningful sounds and had pretty good bodily sensations.

How had Sharpie known he was now acting like an eighteen-month-old? That was easy, too. We knew hundreds of well eighteen-month-olds. Eighteen-month-olds could walk, they could say about eighteen words, they could pick up tiny objects between thumb and forefingers. They could do those motor things because they could converge their vision. They could understand many words and they could feel the third dimension.

That's what she had done. That's really all she'd done.

I looked at my drawing board on which I had lettered

"THE DEVELOPMENTAL PROFILE"

I was ready to begin.

In the past we had talked of children only up to a year of age, and

THE DEVELOPMENTAL PROFILE

VII	72 Months
VI	36 Months
V	18 Months
IV	12 Months
III	7 Months
II	2.5 Months
I	Birth

FIGURE 8

we had talked of four significant stages. We now knew that from one year of age until about six years of age, when all the basic human neurological processes were functioning at full efficiency, there were three additional stages.

So, all together there were seven stages in the life of a child, running the full spectrum from birth until all human functions were in place and operating.

Seven stages in the spectrum of brain development just as there were seven colors in the spectrum of visible light.

I drew seven horizontal bands and I lightly sketched in the colors of the spectrum starting at the bottom. Red, orange, yellow, green, blue, indigo and violet.

I therefore drew seven horizontal bands, and since I knew from our years of observing children of all kinds the approximate ages at which the normal child moved from stage to stage, I sketched them in as Figure 8.

We knew that a child moved upward through these seven stages as succeedingly higher brain stages came into play. Starting with the medulla at the bottom, I filled them in: medulla, pons, midbrain, and the four significant stages in the development of the human cortex which we called the initial cortex, the early cortex, the primitive cortex and the sophisticated cortex. (See Figure 9.)

Now what were the distinctly human capabilities toward which the human brain had evolved?

What were the functions that distinguished the well child from the hurt child? What were the functions in which our brain-injured children were retarded?

They were walking, talking, writing, reading, hearing (so as to understand speech) and feeling. I assigned a column to each. (See Figure 10.)

However, the functions of walking, talking, writing, reading, understanding and feeling weren't really completely functional until six years of age in an average child, and it was necessary to be able to measure a child at *any* age. Fortunately, we had in our data all the significant steps at the seven critical stages of development for every one of those six functions. We could trace every one of them back to birth.

We were, therefore, not talking simply about the cross-pattern walking, which was complete by six years of age in an average child, but instead about the whole area of human *mobility*, which began at birth with reflex movements of arms and legs.

THE DEVELOPMENTAL PROFILE

VII	72 Mon.	SOPHISTICATED CORTEX
VI	36 Mon.	PRIMITIVE CORTEX
V	18 Mon.	EARLY CORTEX
IV	12 Mon.	INITIAL CORTEX
III	7 Mon.	MIDBRAIN
II	2.5 Mon.	PONS
I	Birth	MEDULLA and CORD

FIGURE 9

THE DEVELOPMENTAL PROFILE

			WALKING	TALKING	WRITING	READING	HEARING	FEELING
VII	72 Mon.	SOPHISTI-CATED CORTEX						
VI	36 Mon.	PRIMITIVE CORTEX						
V	18 Mon.	EARLY CORTEX						
IV	12 Mon.	INITIAL CORTEX						
III	7 Mon.	MIDBRAIN						
II	2.5 Mon.	PONS						
I	Birth	MEDULLA and CORD						

FIGURE 10

We were not talking simply about the talking in complete sentences, which was complete by six years of age in an average child, but instead about the whole of human *language,* which began at birth with one reflex birth cry.

We were not talking simply about using the hands to write language, which the average child is able to do by six years of age, but instead about the whole of human *manual competence,* which begins at birth with the grasp reflex.

We were not talking simply about the human ability to read, which is complete in the average child at six years of age, but about the whole area of human *visual competence,* which begins at birth with a light reflex.

We were not talking simply about the human ability to understand complete sentences through the ear, which is complete in the average child by six years of age, but instead of the whole area of human *auditory competence,* which begins at birth with the startle reflex.

We were not talking simply about the human ability to understand what an object was by feel alone, which is complete in an average child by six years of age, but the entire area of human *tactile competence,* which begins at birth with a number of skin reflexes such as the Babinski.

So I could actually draw the Developmental Profile with six vertical columns from birth to six years of age and give them their larger names. (See Figure 11.)

Now I knew I had what I'd been dreaming about for six years. I finally had my tool. I did not know the precise details, but I saw the pattern with utter and complete clarity.

In my seven layers and six columns I now had forty-two blocks. Each of them was as important as every other because one needed to have every one of them to be neurologically normal.

The seven horizontal bands were for the seven critical ages. The six vertical columns divided three and three. There were three motor columns, each with its seven squares, and three sensory columns, each again divided into the seven critical ages. (See Figures 12 and 13.)

Now I had a picture of a well child's schema of neurological growth. I had forty-two squares each with the age at which the function occurred.

What I had actually come to was a means of determining a child's precise *neurological age* instead of his mere chronological age.

THE DEVELOPMENT PROFILE

			WALKING	TALKING	WRITING	READING	UNDER-STANDING LANGUAGE	IDENTIFYING by FEEL
VII	SOPHISTI-CATED CORTEX	72 Mon.						
VI	PRIMITIVE CORTEX	36 Mon.						
V	EARLY CORTEX	18 Mon.	MOBILITY COMPETENCE	LANGUAGE COMPETENCE	MANUAL COMPETENCE	VISUAL COMPETENCE	AUDITORY COMPETENCE	TACTILE COMPETENCE
IV	INITIAL CORTEX	12 Mon.						
III	MIDBRAIN	7 Mon.						
II	PONS	2.5 Mon.						
I	MEDULLA and CORD	Birth	REFLEX MOVEMENT	REFLEX BIRTH CRY	GRASP REFLEX	LIGHT REFLEX	STARTLE REFLEX	BABINSKI REFLEX

FIGURE 11

THE MOTOR COLUMNS

MOBILITY	LANGUAGE	MANUAL COMPETENCE
Using a leg in a skilled role which is consistent with the dominant hemisphere	Complete vocabulary and proper sentence structure	Using a hand to write which is consistent with the dominant hemisphere
Walking and running in complete cross pattern	2000 words of language and short sentences	Bimanual function with one hand in a dominant role
Walking with arms freed from the primary balance role	10 to 25 words of language and two-word couplets	Cortical opposition bilaterally and simultaneously
Walking with arms used in a primary balance role most frequently at or above shoulder height	Two words of speech used spontaneously and meaningfully	Cortical opposition in either hand
Creeping on hands and knees, culminating in cross-pattern creeping	Creation of meaningful sounds	Prehensile grasp
Crawling in the prone position culminating in cross-pattern crawling	Vital crying in response to threats to life	Vital release
Movement of arms and legs without bodily movement.	Birth cry and crying	Grasp reflex

FIGURE 12

THE SENSORY COLUMNS

VISUAL COMPETENCE	AUDITORY COMPETENCE	TACTILE COMPETENCE
Reading words using a dominant eye consistent with the dominant hemisphere	Understanding of complete vocabulary and proper sentences with proper ear	Tactile identification of objects using a hand consistent with hemispheric dominance
Identification of visual symbols and letters within experience	Understanding of 2000 words and simple sentences	Description of objects by tactile means
Differentiation of similar but unlike simple visual symbols	Understanding of 10 to 25 words and two-word couplets	Tactile differentiation of similar but unlike objects
Convergence of vision resulting in simple depth perception	Understanding of two-words of speech	Tactile understanding of the third dimension in objects which appear to be flat
Appreciation of detail within a configuration	Appreciation of meaningful sounds	Appreciation of gnostic sensation
Outline perception	Vital response to threatening sounds	Perception of vital sensation
Light reflex	Startle reflex	Babinski reflex

FIGURE 13

If the ages I had assigned to each of these functions were true, I had my invaluable tool. If the ages I had assigned were not true but only approximations, I had only to dig into the data and refine my approximations.

I'm sure everyone has experienced at least once in life that hugely satisfying feeling of knowing without any shadow of a doubt that he is absolutely right about something even before all the facts are assembled. It isn't something that happens often, but it is such a magnificent feeling that one doesn't need it often. It was the way I felt at that moment. I *knew* and would have staked my life on it.

Now instead of merely measuring a child's chronological age I could measure six neurological ages (one in each of the areas), and then I could assign him an overall neurological age. What's more, others could use the same tool with reasonable certainty of getting the same results.

As an example, if we are measuring mobility in a child with a chronological age of two years, we know that he should be able, if he is average, to walk with his arms freed from the primary balance role, as the mobility column shows for an eighteen-month-old, but not yet to be able to walk and run in cross pattern as a thirty-six-month-old is able to do.

Now, let us suppose that in actuality he is only taking his first steps, as the mobility column shows a twelve-month-old to be able to do. Then his neurological age in mobility would be only twelve months, or half of his chronological age.

Or take language. Suppose this same two-year-old had only two words of speech. This being the level of language function of a normal twelve-month-old, we are once again looking at a neurological age of only half his chronological age.

Let us suppose we go on to record his level of achievement in the other four functions, using the other four columns. We might come up with the following rather precise picture of this child.

Chronological Age			Neurological Age
24 months	—	mobility	— 12 months
24 months	—	language	— 12 months
24 months	—	manual competence	— 10 months
24 months	—	visual competence	— 15 months

| 24 months | — | auditory competence | — | 18 months |
| 24 months | — | tactile competence | — | 10 months |

Chronological age: 24 months   Aggregate neurological age: 77 months
Divide by 6
Over-all neur. age: 12.8 months

With this new tool I saw at once that I could do a dozen vital things that I had never been able to do before. Many of the things I could do with the Developmental Profile did not become clear to me for several more years, but among the things I knew even then were these.

1. Now that I could measure a child's precise neurological age as well as his precise chronological age, I could tell who needed us and who did not. If his neurological age was below his chronological age, he needed us.

2. Closing the gap between his neurological age and his chronological age in each column was our assignment.

3. When his neurological age in each column reached his chronological age in each column, we had done our job.

4. By comparing his initial neurological age with his initial chronological age, I could determine his average *rate* of growth up to the time he saw us. Take, for example, another child, three years old, but operating at only a one-year level:

Neurological age: *12 months*
Chronological age: *36 months*   = rate of growth ⅓ normal

5. By comparing his increase in neurological age with his increase in chronological age at any time after treatment began, I could determine whether a child's development was improving significantly. For example, the child cited above might have been measured again after a year on the program with the following results.

Neurological age: *30 months*—increase in neurological age:
18 months
Chronological age: *48 months* —increase in chronological age:
12 months

Present rate of growth 1.5 x normal
Previous rate of growth ⅓ normal
Increase in rate of growth 4.5 x previous rate of growth.

In such a case it would be clear that *something* had made a significant improvement in his rate of growth. (Theoretically, the improvement could have been the result of chance or misdiagnosis rather than our programs of treatment, but after our case histories climbed into the hundreds and later into the thousands, we allowed ourselves to credit the programs.)

6. By comparing the new rate of growth with how far he has to go to reach normal, we can determine whether the new rate of growth, if it continues, will reach normal in a reasonable length of time.

Continuing with the same child, we can see that his growth has jumped from a rate at which he was falling further behind every year to a rate at which he is catching up. He is presently gaining neurological maturity at the rate of 18 months in an elapsed period of 12 months. If this rate of growth continues another year, his quotient of neurological age over chronological age (NA/CA) will be 48/60. Two years hence it will be 66/72. Thus, in less than three years more he will reach full neurological maturity (72 months—no one, regardless of age, can score higher than 72 months of neurological age on this scale). That would seem to be an entirely acceptable rate of progress. If, on the other hand, such a projection showed that his new rate of growth would require ten additional chronological years (which would make him 16 years of age) to reach neurological maturity (72 months), one would have to carefully consider whether such a course of action was too unrewarding.

7. I could now demonstrate that a child who performs (as a result of brain injury) at a far lower level than other children, does so because of disability and not because of low intelligence.

Although I shall not take the space to discuss it here, I could also demonstrate, simply by looking at a profile with a line drawn across it at a child's chronological age and with six lines drawn across at the child's actual level of performance, whether or not a child was brain-injured; if brain-injured, whether the injury was mild, moderate, severe, profound or complete; whether it was focal or diffuse; whether it was on one side of the brain or on both and at what level of brain the injury existed.

Although I did not know it at the time we would one day be able to use it to measure intelligence, to demonstrate the reason for that I.Q. and, finally, to demonstrate what to do to raise the intelligence. But these are subjects for future books: "The Brain-injured, Brain-damaged, Mentally Retarded, Mentally Deficient, Cerebral-palsied, Emotionally Disturbed, Flaccid, Rigid, Autistic, Epileptic, Athetoid

Child—How to Treat Him at Home" and "Birth to Six—The Genesis of Genius."

But all this was much in the future, and at that moment at my drawing board so long ago I was sublimely happy. Although it was by then after 10 P.M. I *had* to test my idea and my approximations.

I called in the two people I believed had the most actual detailed knowledge of children. Interestingly, they were both nurses. I called Sharpie and I called Hazel. I was sure they would both still be working, and they were. They came at once.

Since Hazel has always known me and my moods and since Sharpie was also an extremely perceptive person, they could see instantly that I was elated.

"You've discovered something and it's something very important," Hazel said with absolute certainty.

"It has to do with measurement and it's a product of my brilliance," said Sharpie with equal certainty.

"Each of you take a pad and pencil," I said, "and write the answer to questions that I'm going to ask you."

They had begun to catch my sense of elation and they looked at me expectantly.

"A child is just beginning to take his first steps. Write down how old he is."

"A well child?" asked Hazel.

"Yep, a well child."

They both wrote.

"Suppose he wasn't well but instead was brain-injured?" I asked.

"Severely brain-injured?" asked Sharpie.

"Yep."

"Then," she allowed, "he would never walk unless we did something about it."

"Suppose he were mildly brain-injured?"

"He might walk between two and three years of age," said Hazel.

"What did each of you write on your paper for the well child?"

"Twelve months," said Sharpie.

"One year," said Hazel simultaneously.

"Next question: A child is just twelve months old. Write down what he's doing visually."

"A well child?" asked Sharpie.

They both clearly had the picture of what we were doing although they had not yet seen the schema.

"Yes," I said.

We all wrote that a well one-year-old had: (a) a light reflex, (b) outline perception, (c) the ability to see details, (d) could converge his vision and did.

We played the game for an hour with the girls becoming more and more excited as they began to see the ramifications.

"You're comparing the way a child actually behaves . . ." Sharpie began.

"That's called neurological age," I interrupted.

". . . with the age he actually is," finished Sharpie.

"And that's called actual age," guessed Hazel.

"Close but not exactly. It's called chronological age on the Developmental Profile."

"What is a Developmental Profile?" inquired Hazel.

I showed it to them, and they both saw its significance immediately.

We tried one more game.

"If a child cannot crawl, use his hands or say a single word, is he normal?"

"He is if he's a newborn," said Sharpie.

"And if he has a chronological age of ninety-six months?"

"Severely brain-injured."

"And if he has a chronological age of twelve months?"

"Moderately brain-injured."

"And if he's got a chronological age of nine months?"

"Mildly brain-injured."

We talked till daylight.

For many months Dr. Bob, Carl and I discussed the Profile at great length.

We confirmed and reconfirmed the data.

We spent the next twelve years refining the data as we examined more and more hundreds of children.

We are still refining it.

Up to that time our work had been entirely pragmatic in nature no matter how elaborate the theoretical structure upon which it was based. Of course, we had collected large amounts of empirical data, and no clinician in his right mind would sneer at or in conscience ignore empirical data (especially in large quantities). Nonetheless, it was empirical.

With the development of the Profile we could begin to measure, and as a consequence, we could fairly begin to think of ourselves as scientists as well as clinicians.

The Doman-Delacato-Doman Profile has been used to record precise data, to measure, to evaluate and to re-evaluate thousands of children in the United States and tens of thousands of children in Brazil, Argentina, Peru and in dozens of other nations.

In excess of a quarter of a million of the Profile charts have been used in this nation alone.

The Profile is used more widely every day.

A copy of the Profile as it is today is shown following page 128.

20.

CLOSING THE BREAK
IN THE CIRCUIT

As the sixties began, each child was having an individual program prescribed for him, but the factors which those programs had in common were as follows:

1. All children were encouraged to spend a maximum period of time on the floor except when being treated, fed or loved. That time on the floor was spent in the prone position if at level one in the mobility column of the profile. If the child was at a higher level but still unable to crawl properly, he crawled while on the floor. If he was at a higher level but did not creep properly, he crept while on the floor.

2. All children were patterned in truncal patterning, homolateral patterning, cross patterning or cross-pattern walking depending on where the gaps existed in the mobility column or in any other column of the profile.

3. All children were being masked for precisely sixty seconds out of each waking hour so that they would build better chests to cut down on respiratory illnesses and to supply better nutrition to the brain in terms of the oxygen, glucose and trace elements, which are the nutrition of the brain in a clinical sense.

4. All children were being given a language-development program. This emphasized unlimited opportunity to perform at the upper limits of their existing competence. We identified the level at which a child was not yet fully proficient, and gave him opportunity to reinforce that function, as well as unlimited opportunity to embark upon the next higher level.

5. All children were receiving a program of manual-competence development. This aimed to provide unlimited opportunity to perform at both the lowest level on the profile at which they were not yet fully proficient and also at the highest level.

It was more than interesting that in these motor areas (mobility, language and manual competence) a therapist's role *could not be an active one,* since it was clear beyond question that the motor pathways were one-way paths from the brain out, and thus the therapist could in no way affect the brain by use of them. Only the patient could play an active role. All we could do here was to pinpoint the level in each motor column of the Profile at which the patient's function ceased or slowed, and then provide the patient with enormous opportunities to push ahead on his own.

6. Each child was being measured carefully in the visual column of the Profile in order to identify the upper limits of his visual development. He was then given active stimulation aimed at breaking through any barrier to function in the visual neural circuits, at the next higher level.

7. Each child was being measured carefully against the auditory column of the Profile in order to identify the upper limits of his hearing development. He was then given active stimulation aimed at awakening function in the audio neural circuits at the next higher level.

8. Each child was being measured carefully in the tactile column of the Profile in order to identify the upper limits of his tactile competence. He was then given active stimulation aimed at helping him break through to the next higher level.

It now dawned on us that whereas there was *no way* the physical therapist, speech therapist or occupational therapist could reach the brain through the outbound motor pathways of the nervous system, there was an enormously important role for him in reaching them through the inbound sensory pathways.

No wonder therapists had been dejected over the persistent failure of their best efforts. It was as if they had been trying to drive north in the southbound lane of a busy highway. On the other hand, a simple change of lanes—a change to the sensory lanes—might let them progress beyond their fondest hopes. The sensory pathways into the brain through the eyes, ears and skin of the patient were also entirely one-way—but *in.*

Here was revelation indeed for not only had we traditionally tried to put our message *in* through the outward-bound motor pathways instead of through the inward-bound sensory pathways, but in all of my own education in physical therapy I cannot remember any single suggestion that the sensory pathways *might* be used. Except as a neurophysical fact in neurophysiology, neuroanatomy and neuropathology, they were scarcely mentioned.

Not only is it true that we never so much as suspected that we had any responsibility for treating a patient's sensory pathways, I am confident that if someone in, let's say 1955, had suggested that therapy could effectively be administered only in sensory areas, he would have been considered as mad as a hatter.

And this is odd, considering that knowledge of the neural pathways is more than a hundred years old.

How then did we locate the "road closed" signs in the neural pathways in order to be able to concentrate our efforts on that stretch of pathway where the trouble really lay?

It is helpful to look once more at a diagram showing how visual stimulation, auditory stimulation and tactile stimulation enter the brain through the back of the central nervous system to supply the information which the brain needs to supply a motor response, or output, through the front of the central nervous system in terms of mobility, language or manual response. (See Figure 14.)

While all three sensory pathways supply information to the brain and thus to all of the motor pathways, there is a general correspondence between the three pathways described as separate loops.

If tactile pathways are totally destroyed, mobility will be totally destroyed as will manual competence.

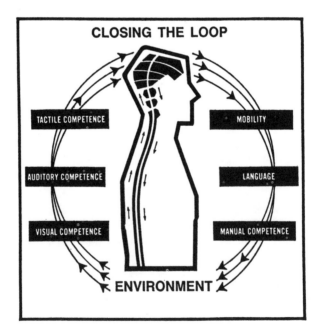

FIGURE 14

If auditory pathways are totally destroyed, language will be virtually destroyed.

If visual pathways are destroyed, manual competence will be greatly interfered with, as will mobility.

If *all* sensory pathways are destroyed entirely, the loop will be broken and the human being will not survive long without extraordinary measures being taken.

If *all* motor pathways are destroyed entirely, the loop will be broken and the human being will not survive long without extraordinary measures being taken.

It is not *possible* to completely destroy all six pathways without destroying the human being.

If these pathways are partially destroyed, there will be partial loss of functions.

Until such a partial or total gap in the loop is found and repaired there will be a mild, moderate, severe, profound or total loss in human walking, talking, writing, reading, understanding or feeling or in several or in all of these human functions.

On the other hand, the brain is not at all the delicate organ we have for so long fancied it to be. It is a tough organ, one of the hardiest in the body, capable of taking grave insult and yet surviving. It would have to be else man would never have survived.

I have three personal friends who each got a bullet through the brain, and each not only survived but survived very nicely. It is worthy of note that none of them are friends of mine as a result of rehabilitation. They are military friends, and I had nothing to do with their rehabilitation. It might be worthwhile to tell the stories of these men.

The first of my friends was an infantry officer commanding a rifle company in combat in Germany very close to where I was doing the same job. He was wounded and unconscious. When he regained consciousness, there was a German soldier standing beside him who asked Bob if he was an American. Upon being told that he was indeed an American, the German soldier removed Bob's helmet, put a pistol to the right side of his head and pulled the trigger—and thus the bullet entered Bob's brain by the right side. Today, a little over twenty years later, Bob has an important job in Washington which he performs in a superior manner. He is as bright as he ever was and is in better physical condition than I am since he has not allowed himself to grow as—well, as stocky as I have.

The second of my friends, also an infantry officer, was wounded in action in Korea by a bullet which went in the back of his skull and emerged in the front. He spent several months in Walter Reed Hospital, primarily, as he points out, because nobody could understand why he didn't have more problems than he had. His own explanation is highly beguiling but may be less than scientifically conclusive. He explains that he has a Swedish father and an Irish mother and that this has given him a very thick Swedish skull and a very small Irish brain which allowed the bullet to pass through his head without touching his brain. Be that as it may, he has gotten his Ph.D. since his brain injury and is also in even better physical condition than I am. Both he and Bob work every day of their lives, and the only co-workers who know that they were severely brain-injured are the ones they have told.

My third friend is the most hurt of all. George was commanding a rifle company in Belgium during the Battle of the Bulge not far from where I was doing the same thing. He was advancing against the enemy through the sub-zero temperature and deep snow when he was hit through the shoulder by a bullet from a machine gun. As he fell, the next round hit him in the front of his skull on the right side of his forehead and came out through the back of his skull. His company, having seen him hit, advanced to find him lying with a bullet through his brain. Infantry combat does not provide time for mourning even one's best friends. His men shed a tear, swore in bitterness, stuck a rifle in the ground with a helmet on top so that the graves registration people could find the company commander's body in the snow, and continued the attack. *Three days later* the burial party found George's body. As they picked it up to place in the truck to be taken for burial, George moved a little bit, so they took him to the hospital instead. The freezing cold had saved his life in a crude form of human refrigeration or *hypothermia* (which Temple Fay had pioneered so brilliantly five years earlier at Temple University Hospital). Since this was accidental hypothermia, the cold that had saved his life had also frozen him, and so, in the hospital, it was necessary to amputate both of George's legs below the hips and to amputate all the fingers as well as the thumb from his right hand. Starting at the bottom, George had no legs, was partially paralyzed on the left side due to the bullet through the right side of his brain, had no fingers nor thumb on his good hand, had a bullet through his left shoulder and a bullet through the right side of his brain.

In those early days of rehabilitation during World War II, methods were not as good as they are today, and George was pretty badly hurt.

George was provided with artificial legs, and during the process of learning how to use them George fell down and broke both hips. Today, two decades later, George has two artificial legs, two surgically pinned hips, is partially paralyzed on the left side, has no fingers or thumb on his right hand and has had bullets through his left shoulder and his right brain. George also walks and works. The last time I saw George personally was when I met him accidentally in a night club in Paris in 1960. George was all right except for the fact that he was having a little trouble balancing. George doesn't always have trouble balancing, but then he isn't always in a night club in Paris, either. I noticed a good many people were having trouble balancing that night, and some a good deal more trouble than George. George had gotten himself from Boston to Paris without any help and, while I haven't seen him since, I am quite confident that he also got himself home again.

Each of these men had a bullet through the brain, each had his brain severely injured, each is a fine, effective human being. George, who functions well but who has several problems which are quite visible, has them because he was frozen rather than because of his brain injury.

As I have said, the brain is a tough organ, but despite the splendid recovery of my three friends, brain injury *can* affect any of the six areas of function mentioned. Let me review the kind of treatment we developed, area by area.

VISUAL COMPETENCE AND BILLY

Billy is thirty-six months old and should therefore be at level VI on the Developmental Profile if he was an average three-year-old. But as you see from his Profile (Figure 15), Billy is unable to perform even at the level of a normal newborn. He does not even have a good light reflex.

We have, then, located the break in the environment-sensory-brain-motor-loop. Now we must close the loop if we are to expect normal performance.

Our goal is to give Billy a *good* light reflex, which is to say, make his pupils contract sharply and promptly when exposed to light and dilate sharply and promptly when exposed to darkness. Billy's light reflex is presently both slow and late in occurring.

Since this break in the loop is in the sensory pathway, the role of patient Billy will be passive and the role of Billy's parents will be

BRAIN STAGE		TIME FRAME	VISUAL COMPETENCE
VII	SOPHISTI-CATED CORTEX	Superior 36 Mon. Average 72 Mon. Slow 108 Mon.	Reading words using a dominant eye consistent with the dominant hemisphere *O*
VI	PRIMITIVE CORTEX	Superior 22 Mon. Average 36 Mon. Slow 70 Mon.	Identification of visual symbols and letters within experience *O*
V	EARLY CORTEX	Superior 13 Mon. Average 18 Mon. Slow 36 Mon.	Differentiation of similar but unlike simple visual symbols *O*
IV	INITIAL CORTEX	Superior 8 Mon. Average 12 Mon. Slow 22 Mon.	Convergence of vision resulting in simple depth perception *O*
III	MIDBRAIN	Superior 4 Mon. Average 7 Mon. Slow 12 Mon.	Appreciation of detail within a configuration *O*
II	PONS	Superior 1 Mon. Average 2.5 Mon. Slow 4 Mon.	Outline perception *O*
I	MEDULLA and CORD	Superior Birth to .5 Average Birth to 1.0 Slow Birth to 1.5	Light reflex *functional*

CHRONOLOGICAL AGE __36__ months

NEUROLOGICAL AGE __0__ months

FIGURE 15

active. Billy's parents will simply stimulate his light reflex over and over again. (The "over and over" part is crucial; we shall often speak of the importance of *frequency, intensity and duration* as basic tactics in our fight to awaken dormant neural pathways.)

Billy gets up at 7:30 and goes to bed at 9 o'clock. We shall have a visual session every half hour, which will allow us twenty-seven sessions each day. Billy's mother takes him into a dark closet which she has prepared with a chair for herself. She sits Billy on her lap and the session begins. She has with her a two-cell flashlight which she shines into Billy's eyes, from a distance of eighteen inches. She shines the light in his eyes for a period of two seconds which she measures by saying slowly, "This is light." She says this aloud—whether Billy understands her or whether he does not. (We use every opportunity for auditory stimulation.) She leaves it turned off for three seconds which she measures by saying (under her breath, this time), "One thousand, two thousand, three thousand." She repeats this entire procedure ten times at each of the twenty-seven sessions. This will mean that Billy will have at least 270 pupillary constrictions daily and at least 270 pupillary dilations daily, and the chances are very strong that Billy's light reflex will improve greatly. As it improves, the chances are very good that he will begin to see outlines (the second block up on the Profile). Thus, we have found the break in the cybernetic loop and we have moved to close it.

AUDITORY COMPETENCE AND MARY

Now let's find an example in the auditory column (also a sensory column). This time we'll take a gap slightly higher in the circuit.

Mary is ten months old and has very large auditory problems. While Billy was in fact functionally blind, Mary is for all practical purposes deaf, but she is not as deaf as Billy was blind. She is also considerably younger than Billy. Her auditory column on the profile looks like this. (See Figure 16.)

Here then is Mary who at ten months of age, if she were an average baby, should be about to enter Stage IV but who is instead functioning at Stage I—the level of a child one month old.

Auditorily, she has a startle reflex which is normal to a newborn. This is to say, if a sudden, loud noise occurs (such as a door slamming) she will immediately jump.

She will jump as often as the sudden noise occurs even if it occurs five times in succession. This is not a product of being afraid, and

BRAIN STAGE		TIME FRAME	AUDITORY COMPETENCE
VII	SOPHISTI-CATED CORTEX	Superior 36 Mon. Average 72 Mon. Slow 108 Mon.	Understanding of complete vocabulary and proper sentences with proper ear ⭕
VI	PRIMITIVE CORTEX	Superior 22 Mon. Average 36 Mon. Slow 70 Mon.	Understanding of 2000 words and simple sentences ⭕
V	EARLY CORTEX	Superior 13 Mon. Average 18 Mon. Slow 36 Mon.	Understanding of 10 to 25 words and two-word couplets ⭕
IV	INITIAL CORTEX	Superior 8 Mon. Average 12 Mon. Slow 22 Mon.	Understanding of two words of speech ⭕
III	MIDBRAIN	Superior 4 Mon. Average 7 Mon. Slow 12 Mon.	Appreciation of meaningful sounds ⭕
II	PONS	Superior 1 Mon. Average 2.5 Mon. Slow 4 Mon.	Vital response to threatening sounds ⭕
I	MEDULLA and CORD	Superior Birth to .5 Average Birth to 1.0 Slow Birth to 1.5	Startle reflex *perfect*

CHRONOLOGICAL AGE __10__ months

NEUROLOGICAL AGE __1__ months

FIGURE 16

Mary is not afraid. It is simply a startle reflex and it is normal to a newborn baby. But Mary is not a newborn baby and should be more advanced auditorily. At Mary's age (and at any age beyond four months) her response should be different to a sudden unexpected noise. It should be different in two ways: first, she should jump and *be frightened* since sudden, loud noises may actually pose a threat to her life (house caving in—earthquake, etc.) and, second, she should not jump or be frightened by subsequent repetitions of the noise since she does not, in fact, find herself threatened by those noises. This second level in the auditory pathway is no longer reflex in nature. It is a vital response to threatening sounds.

While Mary has a true startle reflex, she does not have a vital response to threatening sounds; here is the break in the loop in Mary's case. This will virtually destroy the entire auditory-language loop and will cause large problems to the entire environment-sensory-brain-motor-environment loop.

Since this is a sensory pathway rather than a motor pathway, the parents' role will again be active rather than passive while the baby's role will be passive rather than active.

Let's suppose that Mary wakes at 7 A.M. and is put to bed at 7 P.M. Mother will stimulate her auditorily every waking half hour, which will give her twenty-four sessions a day. Mother will do so by unexpectedly banging two blocks of wood together just behind Mary's head. She does so ten times at three-second intervals in each of the twenty-four sessions. This will give Mary two hundred and forty threatening sounds daily and will require thirty seconds out of each half hour twenty-four times a day for a total of 720 seconds, or twelve minutes.

Since Mary *does* have a startle reflex and does *not* have a vital response to threatening sounds, the result, at first, will be that Mary has two hundred and forty startle reflexes daily. Since this is perhaps one hundred or two hundred or three hundred times as many opportunities for startle reflex as the environment would normally provide, and since moving to each higher brain level of function is the result of brain growth—which is, in turn, a product of the number of times one has the opportunity to use his *present* level of brain function—our hope is that Mary will soon change. Pretty soon we expect that she will *not* jump ten times if the sound is repeated ten times in a row; she will jump perhaps only nine times, and then only eight, and then only seven, and so on. As the number of times Mary startles at repeated noises reduces, Mary will begin not only to startle but also to be afraid and to cry. It is proper to be frightened by a sudden, loud, unexpected noise. Mary has now arrived at Stage II on the auditory pathway and should now begin spontaneously to re-act not only to threatening noises but to other meaningful sounds (such as laughter) as well. If she does not do so spontaneously she will need stimulation at Stage III as well.

Mary's mother has found the break in the cybernetic loop, and she has moved to fill it in.

TACTILE COMPETENCE AND SEAN

The third function to be considered is tactility—the most ignored of all of the sensory functions and one that is vital to movement itself.

Let's consider the case of Sean who is six years old but who is awkward both in walking and in manual competence. We find him to be extremely low in the tactile column of the Profile for a boy who is beginning to read. His tactile column looks like this. (See Figure 17.)

If Sean were an average six-year-old, he should be performing at Stage VII. Because Sean is hurt, we find him instead performing suc-cessfully at Stage I. He has normal superficial reflexes such as the Babinski. He also has normal perception of vital sensation at Stage II, which is to say that he is aware of being burned, being frozen or being physically damaged; however, he has sub-normal ability to feel at the level of Stage III. This is the level of a normal five-month-old. We have found the gap in the circuit for Sean.

Stage III is the ability to appreciate gnostic sensation. It is the ability to "know" meaningful sensations at a more subtle level than at the mere survival level of knowing that one is being burned to death, frozen to death or torn to death. Where Stage II deals with the crude but vital perception of *cold,* Stage III deals with the appreciation of *cool.* Where Stage II deals with the crude but vital perception of *hot,* Stage III deals with the appreciation of *warm.* Where Stage II deals with the crude but vital perception of being cut, crushed or beaten, Stage III deals with the appreciation of being stroked, rubbed or massaged.

Sean deals poorly at Stage III and only dimly appreciates warm, cool and other gnostic sensations.

Since tactility is a sensory pathway, his mother's role will again be active. Mother will give Sean tactile stimulation.

Since Sean is older than the other two children we have examined,

BRAIN STAGE		TIME FRAME	TACTILE COMPETENCE
VII	SOPHISTI-CATED CORTEX	Superior 36 Mon. Average 72 Mon. Slow 108 Mon.	Tactile identification of objects using a hand consistent with hemispheric dominance O
VI	PRIMITIVE CORTEX	Superior 22 Mon. Average 36 Mon. Slow 70 Mon.	Description of objects by tactile means O
V	EARLY CORTEX	Superior 13 Mon. Average 18 Mon. Slow 36 Mon.	Tactile differentiation of similar but unlike objects O
IV	INITIAL CORTEX	Superior 8 Mon. Average 12 Mon. Slow 22 Mon.	Tactile understanding of the third dimension in objects which appear to be flat O
III	MIDBRAIN	Superior 4 Mon. Average 7 Mon. Slow 12 Mon.	Appreciation of gnostic sensation *functional*
II	PONS	Superior 1 Mon. Average 2.5 Mon. Slow 4 Mon.	Perception of vital sensation *perfect*
I	MEDULLA and CORD	Superior Birth to .5 Average Birth to 1.0 Slow Birth to 1.5	Babinski reflex *perfect*

CHRONOLOGICAL AGE __72__ months

NEUROLOGICAL AGE __5__ months

FIGURE 17

he wakes up at seven o'clock in the morning but doesn't go to bed until ten at night. Sean, therefore, has fifteen waking hours and therefore thirty half hours during which a few minutes can be devoted to tactile stimulation.

Sean's mother gets two pans big enough to hold both of Sean's hands. In one pan she puts warm water and in the other she puts cool water. First she sees that Sean puts his hands in the warm water and holds them there for five seconds while she instructs him to look at his hands and reminds him that the water is warm but not hot. She sees that he then removes his hands from the warm water and plunges them directly into the cool water for five seconds while she again directs that he look at his hands and again she tells him that this water is cool but not cold. After five such cycles requiring a little less than a minute in all, she empties the water from the pan. She now massages each of his hands for a full minute, explaining to him that this feels pleasant and instructing him to watch the massaging. She then puts fresh warm water in one pan and fresh cool water in the other pan and repeats the dipping process five times, thus using about five minutes of each half hour of his waking day.

Sean is receiving cool stimulation three hundred times per day (ten immersions—thirty times a day) and warm stimulation three hundred times per day as well as thirty one-minute massages on each hand per day. If one depended on the accidents of environment for this experience we would find that he might be exposed to warm and cool half a dozen times a day and the massage not at all. Thus, Sean's mother provides him in each day with the sensory experiences he might normally have in sixty days.

By so doing, she is providing greatly expanded sensory stimulation. With any luck, his sensory pathway of tactility will begin to develop and as it does he will come to appreciate gnostic (knowing) sensation fully. When he does, he will begin to be able to deal with the third dimension in a tactile sense, which is Stage IV in the tactile pathway.

Sean's mother has thus found and moved to fill in the break in the loop.

By the end of the nineteen-fifties we were closing such breaks with a good deal of regularity, and while we understood what we were doing and what was happening to the kids, we were still reasonably inarticulate as to *why* it was happening—although it was clear that what was happening was good. Very good.

In the cases we have discussed so far, mother has taken an active role and the child a passive role. It is possible for mother to feed visual, auditory and tactile information into her son's brain, even against his will.

She can *not*, on the other hand, walk for him, talk for him or write for him. These things he must, in the end, do for himself. If we find a break in these three motor pathways, we can only provide every opportunity for the child himself to perform these functions. We must do this with great energy, enthusiasm, patience and ingenuity.

Strangely, although everyone had always considered that a child who could not walk or talk or use his hands *must* naturally have his injury in motor areas of the brain (after all, walking, talking and using the hands are motor functions), we found that in the vast majority of brain-injured children this only *appeared* to be the case. In truth we found that the break in the loop is far more commonly on the sensory side of the loop than it is on the motor side of the loop. This did not mean, of course, that his motor skills would test higher than his sensory skills.

When one has time to think about it, it becomes embarrassingly obvious that a child is *never* higher on the motor side of the Profile than he is on the sensory side, and indeed quite the reverse is almost always the case. Almost invariably the child is considerably higher on the sensory side of the Profile than he is on the motor side. Even a little loss of function on the sensory side usually implies more loss of function on the motor side. Indeed, how could it be otherwise? How, for instance, could a child put out normal language on the motor side if he did not take in language on the auditory column on the sensory side of the Profile, which is after all nothing more than the other side of the same coin?

How could a child move his body from place to place (on the mobility column on the motor side of the Profile) if he could not *feel* his body and so did not know where his body was now (in the tactile column on the sensory side of the Profile)?

How could a child write a language (in the manual-competence column on the motor side of the Profile) if he could not see what that language looked like (on the visual column on the sensory side of the Profile)?

The sum of the sensory side of the Profile always equals (and in the vast majority of cases it exceeds) the sum of the mobility side of the Profile. For indeed we cannot possibly put out what we have not somehow taken in.

We're ready now to consider what gaps *can* occur in children on the motor side of the Profile and how we may fill them in and thus close the loop.

The first column on the motor side of the Profile is mobility, so let's consider the case of Lisa who at four years old did not speak and had visual problems. She appeared to be bright and intelligent although she had no ways of proving that beyond the brightness of her eyes and the fact that she smiled and frowned and cried at appropriate times.

The mobility column in her profile looked like this. (See Figure 18.)

If she were average, she should be at Stage VI on the mobility column. Instead, Lisa had successfully reached only that level in the Profile (Stage I) where we would expect to find an average one-month-old infant.

Lisa's mother was a high school graduate and Dad was a shop foreman. Lisa's parents had been told over and over again that Lisa was a vegetable and an idiot and that she should be "put away before you get to love her." Her dad pointed out that it was already too late since he had already loved her for four years and that her mother had loved her long before she had known whether Lisa was going to be a boy or girl. In any event, by the time she was four years old Lisa's family had discovered The Institutes.

Lisa was given a program of visual, auditory and tactile stimulation of the brain with increased frequency, intensity and duration. In between her other periods of stimulation she was to be placed in the prone position on the clean linoleum-covered floor of a warm room so that she might have virtually unlimited opportunity to discover how to move her arms and legs in such a way as to push herself forward and crawl. Thus, Lisa's parents were giving her opportunity to crawl and, thus, to fill in the mobility gap. It is an obviously reasonable approach to mobility, and in a high number of children it works.

After two months of intensive treatment by her parents (nine hours a day, seven days a week), Lisa was a different child, and when she returned to The Institutes for her first re-evaluation her parents were extremely enthusiastic and very grateful. Her understanding of language was now beyond question. She could use her hands for the

BRAIN STAGE		TIME FRAME	MOBILITY
VII	SOPHISTI- CATED CORTEX	Superior 36 Mon. Average 72 Mon. Slow 108 Mon.	Using a leg in a skilled role which is consistent with the dominant hemisphere O
VI	PRIMITIVE CORTEX	Superior 22 Mon. Average 36 Mon. Slow 70 Mon.	Walking and running in complete cross pattern O
V	EARLY CORTEX	Superior 13 Mon. Average 18 Mon. Slow 36 Mon.	Walking with arms freed from the primary balance role O
IV	INITIAL CORTEX	Superior 8 Mon. Average 12 Mon. Slow 22 Mon.	Walking with arms used in a primary balance role most frequently at or above shoulder height O
III	MIDBRAIN	Superior 4 Mon. Average 7 Mon. Slow 12 Mon.	Creeping on hands and knees, culminating in cross pattern creeping O
II	PONS	Superior 1 Mon. Average 2.5 Mon. Slow 4 Mon.	Crawling in the prone position culminating in cross pattern crawling O
I	MEDULLA and CORD	Superior Birth to .5 Average Birth to 1.0 Slow Birth to 1.5	Movement of arms and legs without bodily movement perfect

CHRONOLOGICAL AGE __48__ months

NEUROLOGICAL AGE __1__ months

FIGURE 18

first time. Her personality had blossomed and she now demonstrated a keen sense of humor. Lisa had done beautifully in her first two months of treatment. There was only one problem. Despite many hours daily on the floor Lisa still could not move.

A new program was designed for this new little girl. She was assigned even more time on the floor in the prone position to expand her opportunity to learn to crawl.

When, two months later, Lisa returned for her second revisit her parents were absolutely enraptured with her very obvious progress. Lisa was beginning to talk and now had seven words of language, and although she was only a little past four years of age, Lisa could read words. Now the world could see what Mom had always believed, that despite her staggering disabilities, Lisa was a bright little girl. Only one thing marred their joy. Lisa, despite many, many hours of opportunity could not crawl.

When one watched Lisa on the floor straining every muscle in her body to move, it was obvious that she was using as much effort to move as Dad would have used to move a piano single-handed. It was equally obvious that Lisa had not the faintest notion how to go about moving. Giving Lisa the opportunity to crawl had not been enough.

It is enough for a perfectly well infant. When a well infant is put on the floor in the belly-down position, he does not know how to crawl either, but he is tiny and his arms and legs move freely. He has an additional thing going for him. There is built into his ancient genetic memory a command for his arms and legs to move in a propulsive pattern, and when his body is face down, they will do so. Since he weighs almost nothing, these movements will occasionally result in pushing him forward. When this has happened by accident over and over again, the baby discovers which movements have that effect and which do not. He then discovers how the movements that push him forward *feel* as distinguished from how the movements that do not push him forward *feel*. He finally discovers how to *purposely* reproduce those motions that push him forward and how to synchronize them with each other into a pattern. This may be homologous, homolateral or cross pattern. In any case, he is now crawling; this is the way babies have learned to move since time began for man. And so powerful is that ancient command to move at all costs and at whatever effort, that even the majority of brain-injured children will move to the rhythm of that ancient beat. Just as Robert Ardrey opted to call his book about the development of man *The Territorial Imperative,* I am sure he would call this "The Movement Imperative." It is built-in, basic and almost omnipresent. For even the severely brain-injured child, the mere opportunity to be on the floor is usually enough.

For some severely brain-injured children, however, mere opportunity is not enough (because of the severity, or the precise location of their brain injury or because they are no longer tiny and no longer almost weightless). Lisa was one of these.

It was not merely that trying to move was a prodigious effort for Lisa nor was it merely that moving her arms and legs had not taught Lisa how to move her body forward. What Lisa had learned was far worse than that. Lisa *had* tried to use her arms and legs to push her body forward and she had not succeeded. Lisa had actually learned that arm and leg movement was *not* what caused her body to move forward. Unhappily what she had learned was not true—but from her own experience she had every right to believe it was true.

It was time for Lisa to see and to feel the truth and the inclined plane was the way to demonstrate that truth to her. Although it now seems to me to be as obvious as the nose on my face, it had not seemed obvious to me thirty years earlier and it had taken me until 1945 to develop the idea.

The purpose of the inclined plane, we explained to Lisa's parents, was to give Lisa a chance to learn that there *was* a relationship between her arms, legs and movement. (The opposite to what her own abnormal experience had taught her.)

First they were to take a piece of plywood with one smooth side. It was to be eight feet long and thirty inches wide. It was to have two sides, eight inches high, fastened along the long axis of the plywood so as to create a long chute open at both ends. (See Figure 19.)

Now if we should put Lisa in that chute with her feet at one open end and with her head toward the far end, and if we should lift one end of that chute up in the air high enough to create a sliding board effect, it is obvious that Lisa would slide down it whether she wanted to or not.

Her parents had to find the precisely perfect elevation point for Lisa. That is, the precise point (generally between three and four feet off the floor at the lifted end) at which Lisa, lying still, will not move at all but where, if she makes the slightest movement of arm or leg, however random, she will slide forward a little bit. At that precise point she will stop and not move forward again until she again moves an arm or a leg. This will not have to occur too many times

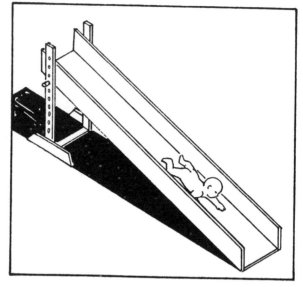

FIGURE 19

before Lisa will discover the clear-cut relationship between movement of arms and legs and getting the body from one place to another.
At that moment we shall have accomplished a very large objective. Lisa will know the secret of crawling. Thus, we will have given
Lisa opportunity to move and to close the loop in this area of
mobility.

Our role here is passive and the child's role is active, but we have
clearly *helped* her to be active.

We also have another objective for Lisa and that is that Lisa should
like moving and conclude that moving is a good and rewarding thing
to do. To accomplish this latter objective, we gave Lisa's parents
the following instructions:

1. The inclined plane must always be at the angle that makes
movement easy and pleasant for Lisa.

2. Once Lisa is put on the inclined plane she must know that the
only way out is at the other end and that this is inevitable and that
fussing will not get her out if she happens to feel irritable.

3. If it takes her longer than one minute to get to the bottom, the
board is too low and should be raised.

4. When she gets to the bottom she is to be instantly picked up,
praised honestly and profusely for her great accomplishment. In

short, Mommy is to make clear to Lisa the joy she herself feels at watching her daughter move at last. Lisa is to be rewarded with love, with praise and with a gift of favorite food, perferably something which she loves but shouldn't have. There should not be the slightest doubt in anybody's mind that this is a special and most wonderful occasion.

5. Once she has reached the bottom and has had her praise and reward she is not to be put back in again for at least a half hour lest Lisa decide that the reward for doing the job well was to have to do it again. By dealing in such a way with Lisa we can arrange for her to say to herself, "Every time Mommy puts me in this thing and I move my arms and legs I move myself forward easily and quickly. What's more, when I finish that exciting business the old girl thinks I'm great and I get loved, praised and bribed with my favorite cookies and I'll be delighted when she puts me back in again because I love to move."

They may not be the exact words that Lisa will use but that will be the right music.

Lisa's family understood and went home to make her inclined plane. Two days later they called us to announce that Lisa had just come down her chute for the first time. They were excited, to put it mildly. Lisa had taken to it like a duck to water. As her dad put it, "You could see her discovery of her arms and legs on her face. When she realized that every time an arm or leg moved she moved forward a little, you could see the surprise and pleasure on her face. You could see her saying to herself as she looked at her own arms and legs, 'Holy Mackerel! That's what they're for.' It was wonderful to watch her."

We then explained to Lisa's parents what they had to do next.

Next they must add to Lisa's opportunity to move on a flat surface by lowering the height of the high end of the board. They were to lower it a very small amount and keep it at the new height until Lisa could swarm down it as easily as she had at the greater angle. They were never to lower it again until she could crawl its length as easily as she had before.

And so they were to proceed until the board was flat on the ground and Lisa was crawling.

They never actually got to that. Before they had gotten it to flat Lisa had crawled down the board and had just continued to crawl across the floor. They had succeeded. Lisa could crawl. They had filled in the gap in the loop at Stage II and Lisa was a moving child.

She was firmly entrenched on the ancient road to walking and all Lisa's mother had done was to give her opportunity, but she had done so with imagination and with love.

Chris was four years and two months old and as bright as a button, but Chris couldn't say one word of English for all of the fact that he clearly understood all that anyone said to him (and, for that matter, what the grownups said to each other). He had been paralyzed when we had seen him originally at three, but he had learned to crawl and now he could creep on hands and knees. He was on his way to walking, but for all of that, as I have said, he couldn't speak one word of English and the language column on his Profile looked like this. (See Figure 20.)

Chris, being fifty months old, should, if he were an average four-plus child, be at Stage VI in language.

Instead Chris was at Stage III. At birth he'd had the reflex birth cry (Stage I). He then learned to cry in such a way that his mother would come (and come running) if he cried in such a way as to indicate that he was in great pain. This was Stage II.

He was now operating at Stage III, meaning that he could make all sorts of meaningful sounds and mother could tell whether he was happy, bored, excited, hungry, content, irritated and a number of other things just by listening to the sounds he made even when she was in another room from him and couldn't see him. He was, however, fifty months old, and should have been able to do all this at seven months.

There was absolutely no question that Chris could hear and understood all he heard. If you didn't want him to understand you had to spell and some words it wasn't even safe to spell, like *bed* and *bath* both of which he hated.

Still Chris had no word of English, and only two sounds that were wordlike. He said something that sounded like "may" and something that sounded like "uhh." It was decided to use these two sounds to establish two words—*Mom* and *up*.

Chris woke up at 7:30 A.M. and went to bed at 9 o'clock, which gave him thirteen and a half waking hours or twenty-seven half-hour periods.

Chris and his mother would have twenty-seven five-minute language-opportunity periods during the day.

BRAIN STAGE		TIME FRAME	LANGUAGE
VII	SOPHISTI-CATED CORTEX	Superior 36 Mon. Average 72 Mon. Slow 108 Mon.	Complete vocabulary and proper sentence structure O
VI	PRIMITIVE CORTEX	Superior 22 Mon. Average 36 Mon. Slow 70 Mon.	2000 words of language and short sentences O
V	EARLY CORTEX	Superior 13 Mon. Average 18 Mon. Slow 36 Mon.	10 to 25 words of language and two-word couplets O
IV	INITIAL CORTEX	Superior 8 Mon. Average 12 Mon. Slow 22 Mon.	Two words of speech used spontaneously and meaningfully O
III	MIDBRAIN	Superior 4 Mon. Average 7 Mon. Slow 12 Mon.	Creation of meaningful sounds *perfect*
II	PONS	Superior 1 Mon. Average 2.5 Mon. Slow 4 Mon.	Vital crying in response to threats to life *perfect*
I	MEDULLA and CORD	Superior Birth to .5 Average Birth to 1.0 Slow Birth to 1.5	Birth cry and crying *perfect*

CHRONOLOGICAL AGE __50__ months
NEUROLOGICAL AGE __7__ months

FIGURE 20

They went to the most comfortable arm chair in the house, away from all commotion. Mother began each session by explaining to Chris that she knew that he was a very smart boy but she also knew that he had trouble talking.

She then explained that they were going to take the sound "may," and in order to make that *Mom*—herself—anytime he ever said "may" she would respond as if he had said "Mom." She also explained that they would take the sound "uhh," which he could already say, and use that to mean "up," so that anytime he said "uhh" she would come and pick him up. She also explained that this was really the exact way that everyone else had learned to talk and that almost everywhere in the world mothers were called "Mom" or "Ma." (This is no coincidence but is a result of the fact that the "m" sound is one of the first sounds a baby can make and that mothers the world over have always said, "You bet, that's me.")

Then mother and Chris would spend the rest of the five minutes trying. Every time Chris said "may" or anything like it, mother would say, "Yes, Chris, what is it?" Any time Chris said "uhh," mother would say, "Yes, Chris," and then she would pick him up.

Chris enjoyed the game and tried very hard. Chris's mother never said, "No, Chris, that doesn't sound like 'Mom,' say it again." Instead she always responded every time Chris said any M sound or any U sound. Sometimes Chris forgot and said "may" when he didn't mean "Mom," but his mother always responded any time during the day when he said "may" as if Chris had called her. This made them both laugh. She also picked him up every time he said "uhh."

Within a month Chris came to use the "may" sound only to mean mother and the "uhh" sound only when he wanted to be picked up. In another month the "may" sound had begun to sound a lot like "Mom" and the "uhh" sound a lot like "up." He had also developed some new sounds. Thanks to the other aspects of the program his chest got better (from increased mobility) and his brain functioned better (from the increased oxygen supply to the brain). Chris had progressed to Stage IV in the language column of the Profile and was headed for V.

His mother had found the break in the loop and she had wisely given Chris the opportunity to complete the loop.

MANUAL COMPETENCE AND SUZIE

Suzie was two and a half years old and had staggering problems. She had been a perfectly healthy baby up until eleven months of age at which time she had had a very high temperature for twenty-four hours and a severe encephalitis. The encephalitis had left Suzie with an almost total lack of function.

Her manual competence column looked like this. (See Figure 21.)

Suzie, who was thirty months old should, if she were average, have been performing at Stage V.

In fact, because she was a very brain-injured little girl as the result of her encephalitis, she could operate only at Stage I in manual competence, which is to say that she had a grasp reflex. This meant that if you put something inside Suzie's clenched fist it would remain clenched in her fist until in moving her arms it would eventually be knocked out.

It wasn't that Suzie could *hold on* to an object as a newborn baby can. It was that, exactly like a newborn baby, she couldn't *let go*. This was Stage I, grasp reflex.

Suzie could *not* perform at Stage II in the manual-competence column. Stage II occurs at 2.5 months of age in an average baby, and it is the function of being able to let go. This stage first occurs in a normal baby as an accident. However, each time the baby happens to let go of something by accident he is (also accidentally) getting the feel of what it is like to let go.

The baby comes finally to feel precisely what all those accidents had in common and learns how to "reproduce the accident" as it were. This is called vital release.

Now it was Suzie's mother's job to give Suzie the opportunity to let go. Nowhere is the example of supplying opportunity more clear than it is in this example of vital release. If you want someone to let go of an object, it is obvious that you have only to put it in his hand until he lets go of it and then to put it back in his hand again.

It is possible that this happens to a one-month-old baby eight or ten times a day since the baby can only let go of an object that some adult has put in his hand.

Suzie's mother had her job cut out for her. She had to supply Suzie in one day with as many opportunities to let go as a well infant gets in fifty or sixty days. She got two half-inch wooden rods (dowels) two inches long which fitted snugly, one in each of Suzie's hands, and every time Suzie lost one of the dowels, her mother put it back in her hand again.

There are more exciting jobs in the world than putting a dowel in a child's hand several hundred times a day, but perhaps there are not many more exciting jobs if a mother sees her paralyzed daughter's hands begin to function as Suzie's hands began to do as a product of

BRAIN STAGE		TIME FRAME	MANUAL COMPETENCE
VII	SOPHISTI-CATED CORTEX	Superior 36 Mon. Average 72 Mon. Slow 108 Mon.	Using a hand to write which is consistent with the dominant hemisphere O
VI	PRIMITIVE CORTEX	Superior 22 Mon. Average 36 Mon. Slow 70 Mon.	Bimanual function with one hand in a dominant role O
V	EARLY CORTEX	Superior 13 Mon. Average 18 Mon. Slow 36 Mon.	Cortical opposition bilaterally and simultaneously O
IV	INITIAL CORTEX	Superior 8 Mon. Average 12 Mon. Slow 22 Mon.	Cortical opposition in either hand O
III	MIDBRAIN	Superior 4 Mon. Average 7 Mon. Slow 12 Mon.	Prehensile grasp O
II	PONS	Superior 1 Mon. Average 2.5 Mon. Slow 4 Mon.	Vital release O
I	MEDULLA and CORD	Superior Birth to .5 Average Birth to 1.0 Slow Birth to 1.5	Grasp reflex *perfect*

CHRONOLOGICAL AGE __30__ months

NEUROLOGICAL AGE __1__ months

FIGURE 21

performing the function over and over and over again. For it is function that creates structure and even in the end the structure of the brain, just as in the evolutionary process man's brain was structured by its functions.

So Suzie's mom had found the break in the loop and had moved to close the circuit. Suzie advanced.

We have looked at one example in each of the six columns of the Profile.

All one does, then, is to check out a child in each of the six columns of the Profile and identify the squares above which the child does not perform normally.

You then start at whatever point the child is sub-normal in his skills and try to give him vastly more opportunities to learn what it is like to perform at the next level.

If the breaks are in any of the three sensory columns, mother simply starts at the lowest break and gives huge amounts of stimulation in each area where the child is falling short.

If the breaks are in any of the three motor columns, mother simply starts at the lowest break and gives the child huge amounts of opportunity to perform at the next level.

So it was with Billy, Mary, Sean, Lisa, Chris and Suzie. Each mother had devoted five or so minutes out of each waking half hour to filling in the particular break in the circuit which has been described. Does it seem like a terribly large amount of time to give, considering the possible pay-off?

Of course as one reflects about it he remembers that each of the children was probably also being patterned for five minutes at least four times a day, seven days a week.

Come to think of it, you may say, don't they also get that masking one minute out of every hour? Now the time is beginning to add up to a great deal of time.

And are you suddenly struck with the fact that few kids are brain-injured in such a way as to be involved in only one column, and most kids are involved in all six columns?

If you multiplied what you do in one column by six columns and then you added . . .

If it occurs to you that if you added it all up there is little time left for performing little tasks like cleaning, cooking, shopping, ironing and other little things, I can only say that I never promised anyone a bed of roses, or for all of that, any bed at all.

A light schedule for a child who has only a reading problem may involve as little as an hour a day. That however would be an exception, and a more typical program would involve eight hours a day. A program might, in point of fact, extend up to thirteen or even more hours a day. Before we have a look at what such a program might be like, let's consider a cardinal point that may not, at first glance, meet the eye. Parents rarely ask for an easier program. When occasionally we think parents need a rest and insist that parents take a break of two months or so, we almost invariably meet the only serious resistance we ever encounter with parents. When a child's entire life is at stake and heroic efforts must be made in a child's behalf, it is not parents who complain about the prodigious efforts that must be made. Rather, it is everyone else who complains in behalf of the parents, whether the parents want such championing or not.

Parents have spent every waking second considering the monumental size of the problem they face. A typical parent comment when faced with a program which would stagger any human being other than a parent is, "What am I going to do if I *don't* do the program?" It isn't that the much maligned parents are so much smarter than anyone else, it is simply that no one else has spent as much time considering the alternatives as they have, and it is also true that no one else loves their child as much as they do.

I am sure that there must, in the world, be parents who do *not* love their children all that much. It is, I guess, just that those parents don't go to the trouble and difficulty of bringing their children to The Institutes. Philadelphia is, after all, very far from all the places in the world that are very far from Philadelphia. Just how far, far is, is highly related to just how important problems seem to each of us.

Parents are in many ways like the staff of The Institutes, and one of these ways is that they spend every waking hour thinking about the problem. They, like we, have often considered the obvious. In this case, the obvious is that while we are not yet smart enough to know *a priori* which kid will win and which kid will lose, it is clear that each kid who is going to win will have to do the things that will help him to function normally "X" number of times. While we have no way of knowing whether "X" is 5,692 times or 56,920 times, it is clear that we can spread "X" out over a lifetime by doing it one time a day for twenty years or by doing it ten times a day for two years. The parents' choice about which of these to do is very clear. I remember a mother to whom I had just given a program that would stagger a marathon runner. "And now," she said, "I hope that while we're home doing this until midnight that all of you will spend whatever spare hours you can find to discover *new* methods that might make Nan better quicker or surer so that the next time we see you, you can *add* them to this program." Bright gal—we will.

Let's look at Nan's program to which Mom wanted to add.

NAN'S PROGRAM

Nan is three years old. She is extremely paralyzed with twisted limbs and much uncontrolled movement of arms, legs, head and face. Nan has a very severe midbrain injury. Her left eye turns in toward her nose. Her face twists every time she tries to talk. Her speech cannot be understood; she cannot crawl, creep or walk. She understands everything said to her and despite her problems is a charming little girl whom everyone loves.

Chronological age	38 months
Neurological age	11.5 months

Time	Activity	Min.
7:30 A.M.	Breakfast (Learning to eat properly)	30
8:00	Patterning ⌗1	5
8:05	Begin Sequence ⌗1	
	Slide	2
	Crawl	3
	Mask	1
	Reading	2
	Visual Stimulation	2
	Crawl	3
	Auditory Stimulation	1
	Tactile Stimulation	3
	Bathroom Training	3
	Language Program	3
	Prehensile Grasp	3
	Mask	1
	Crawl	3
	Total	30
	Time spent moving from place to place	5
	Time spent loving Nan	5
	Grand Total	40

Time	Activity	Min.
8:45	Patterning ⅍2	5
8:50	Sequence ⅍2 (Same as Sequence ⅍1)	40
9:30	Patterning ⅍3	5
9:35	Sequence ⅍3 (Same as Sequence ⅍1)	40
10:05	Sequence ⅍4 (Same as Sequence ⅍1)	40
10:45	Sequence ⅍5 (Same as Sequence ⅍1)	40
11:25	Sequence ⅍6 (Same as Sequence ⅍1)	40
12:05 P.M.	Lunch (Stimulation to eat well)	30
12:35	Sequence ⅍7 (Same as Sequence ⅍1)	40
1:15	Sequence ⅍8 (Same as Sequence ⅍1)	40
1:55	Sequence ⅍9 (Same as Sequence ⅍1)	40
2:35	Sequence ⅍10 (Same as Sequence ⅍1)	40
3:15	Patterning ⅍4	5
3:20	Sequence ⅍11 (Same as Sequence ⅍1)	40
4:00	Patterning ⅍5	5
4:05	Sequence ⅍12 (Same as Sequence ⅍1)	40
4:45	Patterning ⅍6	5
4:50	Sequence ⅍13 (Same as Sequence ⅍1)	40
5:30	Sequence ⅍14 (Same as Sequence ⅍1)	40
6:10	Dinner (Stimulation for mouth and throat)	30
6:40	Sequence ⅍15 (Same as Sequence ⅍1)	40
7:20	Sequence ⅍16 (Same as Sequence ⅍1)	40
8:00	Sequence ⅍17 (Same as Sequence ⅍1)	40
8:40	Sequence ⅍18 (Same as Sequence ⅍1)	40
9:20	End of Nan's Program.	

(Beginning of Nan as a young lady.)

Note: We did as Nan's mother had requested and continued to discover new methods and techniques for Nan. Happily, as we added new things to Nan's program, we were able to drop things she no longer needed.

Parents, then, are perfectly capable of carrying out such staggering programs, and with the help of the entire family they manage to do so sometimes for years on end.

Then how about Nan? Can that twisted, paralyzed, bright-eyed little thing hold up for years of such regimentation? Such a tiny, such a hurt little thing? Of course she does. As a matter of fact, it's quite good for her despite all that might be said by all those who insist that the very best thing we can do for such children's own sake is to expect nothing from them and to pop them forever into a latter-day Bedlam, which would give the Devil nightmares. Those who think it wouldn't, might like to have a glance at a truthful and courageous photo essay called *Christmas in Purgatory* by Burton Blatt and Fred Kaplan (Allyn & Bacon, Publishers). It doesn't attempt to soften the fact, and it couldn't exaggerate it.

It's the people *doing* the patterning who are getting the workout. Most of the things that require Nan's co-operation are by and large the things that are in themselves pleasurable and even joyful. Like reading. No one enjoys reading more or takes greater pride in the accomplishment than a little child. Especially a little hurt child who doesn't have the outdoors competing with reading.

Still, all the things are not as joyful as reading, and the ingenuity of mother and all of her family will be taxed to make them happy functions. The chapter on reading and the chapter on motivation will help in that regard. Still, it's a hard job and cannot always be accomplished by all families. Strangely, it is not so much what the child is like, but instead what the family is like that determines the degree of positive motivation that can be achieved. Basically, family opinion falls into two groups among those who seek the help of The Institutes.

The first group of dedicated families is by far the larger group. They are the families who see the hurt child as an extremely positive factor in family life. These are the families who say, "Everybody adores Joanne. She's the star of our family. We would give anything in the world to fix Joanne, and we are going to fix her, but fixed or unfixed we *want* her. She is an addition to the family, and we don't know what we would do without her." These families see the child as the most marvelous of opportunities and are thrilled to have her.

Hank Viscardi, that determined and marvelous man of stature, who is in a sense one of the founders of rehabilitation, once told me this story.

He once said to his mother, "Mother, why was our family given such a problem as to have me, born with no legs?" His mother said, "Son, when it's time for a crippled child to be born, God has a meeting with all of his advisors and says, 'Where is there a family good enough to be made better by a hurt child?' "

Hank's extraordinary career is not so difficult to explain when one knows that about his mother.

Generally, such families seem able to make even drudgery seem worthwhile for hurt little kids.

The other sort of family we see is equally courageous but less likely to be able to make the program joyous. These families also love the hurt child and are willing also to make tremendous sacrifices for the child. These families, however, are much more likely to see the child as a challenge to the family, perhaps as a cross that the family must bear. Both families love the child; both families are prepared to make heroic sacrifices for him, but these latter are much less likely to be able to motivate him in a positive way.

What then?

Well, eagerly or not eagerly, joyous or not joyous, motivated or not motivated, happily or unhappily, he must be treated if he is to have his chance as a well human being.

There are many things in life all human beings have to do which are, in truth, *not* joyous. Some of them, in fact, are downright drudgery or even painful. But drudgery or painful, they must be done, whether adult or child.

The process that gets such things done is the opposite side of the coin called "motivation." For want of a better name, let's call it "discipline." The best kind of discipline, quite obviously, is the kind called "self-discipline" and self-discipline in a child is every bit as possible as in an adult. In either case, what is needed to achieve self-discipline is an understanding of the goal, and this is often easier to explain to an adult than to a child. It is hard, as an example, to explain to a three-year-old precisely why patterning is a good thing. In any event, one must try even with a hurt three-year-old. The easiest way to explain why patterning is a good thing to a tiny hurt child is to demonstrate to him clearly how happy it makes his family (joyousness), and if this works, it is the best way of all.

If, however, it does not work, it is clear that it must be done. Patterning in a sense is a sort of closed brain surgery, and it is clear that if a child needed brain surgery, or any other kind, no family would dream of leaving the decision to the child. So whatever happens he must be treated if we are to succeed, and we must first try self-discipline. If that works, it is the very best way.

If it does not, we must still see that he is treated, and we must, if necessary, impose discipline.

All human beings require discipline and given an opportunity they will impose it on themselves. Both children and adults are constantly searching to find what the rules are, to find where the edges are which one may not go beyond. We find the need to live within a structure that we know and understand.

I'm confident that if I found myself washed up alone on the shore of a desert island, the first thing I would do after I collected myself would be to say, "Now just what are the rules around here?" And finding none, I should have to make rules of my own lest in the absence of rules of self-discipline I should slide into being less than human. The formalized version of those rules I would impose on myself is called The Law. When we adults find ourselves in the absence of law or structure, we create it. When we find ourselves newly introduced into a situation where rules exist, we seek to find where the edges are—how far we can go.

So too do children. They seek desperately to do so. When Mother puts a child to bed seventeen times and he gets back up eighteen times and is finally walloped, it is not that he has made a mistake. He was demanding to be spanked. He was trying to find where the edges were. In this case he found out. It took eighteen times to find how far he could go.

A child needs discipline in the same way that he needs good food and love and fresh air.

If one is unable to motivate a child in a positive way (which is the very best way), then one must do what must be done.

The simplest, most direct way is the best way.

It is fair to begin by saying to a child, "Johnny, I want you to do this because it is good for you."

If that works, it is the best way.

If that does not work, one should then say, "Johnny, I want you to do this because I am your daddy (mommy) and I have decided you should."

If that works, it is the next best way.

If that doesn't work, the next best way is to say, "Johnny, I want you to do this because if you don't do it, you don't get to watch your favorite TV program (or eat your ice cream or play with the dog or whatever else Johnny likes to do).

If that works, it's the next best way.

If that doesn't work, one should say, "Johnny, I want you to do this because I am bigger than you are and I say so." Now Johnny, no matter how small he is or how hurt he is, is perfectly aware that you are bigger than he is (and so are all the other kids). That's in one sense the only reason any kid ever went to school or ate spinach.

They know we're bigger than they are and often it is enough to remind them of the fact.

If that works, it's the next best way.

If that does not work, one must say, "Johnny, if you don't do that I am going to pop you one."

If that works, it is the next best way.

If that doesn't work, one says, "Johnny, I am about to wham you, and when I'm through belting you, you are going to do it or I am going to wham you again."

It is devoutly to be wished that one never gets to the bottom of the list, but if one does, he must win the battle because by that time the real subject under discussion is which one is the parent and which is the child.

If the child wins such a battle against his parents, then his chance to be well is simply non-existent. If a child fails to get well, it is of very little importance whether the reason is that he has overwhelming pathology, or whether The Institutes' people are not yet capable of solving the problem or whether a parent is unwilling or unable to control the child.

The Institutes' program is an entirely unreasonable program beyond any question.

I know of a dozen or more entirely reasonable programs for brain-injured children. The only problem is that they don't work.

The Institutes' program frequently does work.

I have an idea that a reasonable course of action that does not work is unreasonable.

I also have an idea that an unreasonable program that does often work for brain-injured kids—is reasonable.

The Institutes' program for parents to treat their children is a terrible program, and it gobbles up the lives of everyone concerned with it. It is surely the world's most difficult program.

Of course, every time I think of that I also think about Nan's father who said to me, "There is only one thing in the whole world that is worse than this damned program, and that is having a little girl whom you love who can't do what other kids do. I must say that the worst day on The Institutes' program is better than the best day we had before we began this lousy program."

21.

SO WHAT'S GOING ON IN THE BODY? FUNCTION DETERMINES STRUCTURE

There is a law in nature that is of vital importance to all children and of overwhelming importance to brain-injured children. We have known this law for many years but we have managed somehow to ignore its staggering implications.

At The Institutes it was what we were seeing happening daily to our brain-injured children that forced us to consider this law and what it meant to them.

We were seeing severely brain-injured children arrive with bodies that were almost invariably tiny and sometimes twisted, with shoulders, eyes, mouths and feet that were frequently extremely abnormal, with heads so tiny as to be microcephalic and chests so shallow as to barely supply a breathing apparatus.

When we failed those children, their bodies remained tiny or twisted and so did their backs, hips, eyes, mouths and heads.

But when we succeeded, their bodies became in every way normal.

What is the law that explains this staggering fact? That law states simply that "function determines structure." That law explains why life on earth developed as it did from single-celled life in the primordial tide pools, to fishes, amphibians, mammals and man (phylogeny). That law also explains how human life develops from embryo, to foetus, to newborn (ontogeny).

It is the law that states that weight lifters have huge muscles because they lift weights. It is not that they lift weights because they have big muscles. Function determines structure.

Architects must first know what a building is to be used for before they can draw plans for it because its function will determine the structure.

A baby who is raised for the first year of life in near darkness (as is the case with certain beautiful but pre-Stone Age Xingu tribes with whom we have lived in the interior of Brazil's Mato Grosso) will not develop visually and will retain the visual pathways and competence of a newborn until brought out of the dark hut into light. His lack of visual function will have prevented earlier maturation of his visual pathway.

A child chained since infancy to a bedpost in an isolated attic by a psychotic adult will not develop normal hip sockets since no child is born with true hip sockets but instead actually cuts hip sockets by wearing them into the bone as a result of crawling, creeping and walking. It is not that we walk because we have hip sockets (as we once insisted on believing) but rather that we have hip sockets because we crawl, creep and walk. It is *not* that structure determines function but rather that function (moving) creates structure (hip sockets).

The brain-injured child who cannot move (due to his brain injury) does not develop hip sockets either. Sooner or later someone who does not believe that brain injury is in the brain but instead believes that brain injury is in the legs will send him for hip X-rays and will find that he does not have normal hip sockets. The child will then have orthopedic surgery to create artificial hip sockets. This of course will not work since the child will still not walk for the precise same reason that he did not walk in the first place (brain injury). Not only is it true that function determines structure, but it is equally true that lack of function results in an immature or abnormal structure.

The vast majority of severely brain-injured children are quite tiny in physical size when they are first seen at The Institutes. That is to say, in height, in chest, in head size, in weight, they are, in about 75 per cent of the cases, significantly below average, and 50 per cent are below the smallest 10 per cent of the population, sometimes far, far below. Yet at birth (except for the premature ones) they tended to be at or very near average size. As they get older they become smaller and smaller as compared to children their own age since the lack of physical functioning results in a lack of physical structure. This is exactly the opposite of what happens to the weight lifter. Yet once we start such a child on a program of neurological organization, his rate of growth will change, and often change dramatically. Quite often, in fact, a child who had been growing far slower than normal will suddenly start to grow far faster than normal for his age. Even where he began the program smaller in height, in head and chest circumference, and in weight than 90 per cent of other children in his age bracket, it is commonplace to find him suddenly growing at 250 per cent of the norm for his age.

While this phenomenon appears to be virtually unknown to those who deal with brain-injured children, it is well known to anthropologists and even has a name.

It is called the *catch-up phenomenon.*

This rule says that if a child is seriously ill for any reason, his physical growth will slow down or virtually stop, depending on the illness and its severity. The rule further states that if the child becomes normal, he will then grow faster than his peers to catch up. This, of course, is why it is called the *catch-up phenomenon.*

We see this occurring every day of our lives at The Institutes.

We see also, and it is hardly surprising, that there seems to be a high correspondence between the rate of success and the rate of growth as well as between the ultimate degree of growth and the ultimate degree of success.

That is to say, children who fail to make progress also fail to change in growth rate, children who succeed markedly but not completely, grow markedly but not completely, and children who succeed entirely, grow entirely. While this rule, like all other rules I know, is not invariable, it is almost always so.

This is simply another way of saying that lack of function creates an immature or abnormal structure and that function determines structure.

At The Institutes in Philadelphia, all brain-injured children above the age of eighteen months, except those who are completely blind, are started on a program of reading, using extra-large letters that can be discerned by the immature visual pathways of all except children who are terribly blind or who are unable to discern outlines. (With blind children reading is delayed until they are made able to see outlines.) As a result of this exposure to reading, two things happen.

First: There are many hundreds of brain-injured children two, three or four years old, who can read with total understanding from a few words for some to many, many books for others. I know a few three-year-olds who can read in several languages with complete understanding. The size of the words is reduced as they progress.

Second: Although the world at large believes that children under five are unable to read because their visual pathways are too immature and because their brains are not sufficiently developed, there are hundreds of two-, three- and four-year-olds who are *in fact* reading. What is more, they are brain-injured and what is more, their visual pathways are now *more* highly developed than are the visual pathways of older children who are not brain-injured and who do not read. How can this possibly be explained?

It certainly can *not* be explained on the basis of age, since they are younger, not older, than the children who do not read (normal five-year-olds).

It certainly can *not* be explained on the grounds of some natural superiority. Far from being superior, these children are brain-injured and have often previously been diagnosed as being "mentally retarded." I don't know anyone who believes it is an advantage to be brain-injured.

It can only be explained on the grounds that these children have simply had an *opportunity* to read that other children have not had. That opportunity permitted function, and function in turn created more mature visual pathways since function determines structure.

Very few facts are more important in the treatment of brain-injured children.

The lack of this realization is what has been wrong with the world of brain-injured children in the past. The awareness that function determines structure is one of the important things that is right about the world of brain-injured children today.

22.

SO WHAT'S GOING ON IN THE BRAIN? FUNCTION DETERMINES STRUCTURE

Nobody in the world knows with absolute certainty what is actually going on in the brain and neither do we at The Institutes, but we've got some pretty strong suspicions.

No man in all of history has watched a human brain function in a microscopic cellular sense.

At this moment in history there is simply no way to do so, nor is there likely to be in the predictable future.

Brain function is not alone beyond knowing, but is conceivably beyond understanding even if we knew.

But it is not beyond reasonable surmise or reasonable deduction, and surmise we must in order to explain to the best of our ability those things we see occurring in brain-injured children and in average children as well.

If there is much we do not know about that most incredible of organs, the brain, there is also much that we do know about animal brains in general and human brains in particular.

We know, first of all, that an inflexible rule of nature which has guided medicine, psychology, engineering, architecture and a host of other arts and sciences, is at work no less in the brain than in other mechanisms. That law says that "function determines structure."

It does so no less in the brain than in the body.

Before we look at the neurophysiological evidence that proves this—and proves it beyond the shadow of a reasonable doubt—let's consider those changes we've just discussed which take place in the bodies of children who are being programmed here at The Institutes in Philadelphia.

Let's consider just two of the changes; first, changes in head size among the brain-injured children.

Why, we must ask, do brain-injured children's heads go from growing much slower than average children's heads before treatment begins, to growing two or even three times faster than well children's
heads after treatment commences?

It has been a moot question up to now as to whether skulls grow
to accommodate the brain or whether the brain was simply restricted
to the size that the skull permitted it to be. With the exception of a
very, very small group of children who have a premature closing of
the fontanels (which are the soft spots on top of infant heads), it
would now appear that it is the skull which is forced to grow to accommodate the brain.

We are now seeing skulls growing not only far beyond the rate at
which they are supposed to grow, but far beyond the time when they
are supposed to have stopped growing.

In fact, one analysis of 278 case histories of consecutively admitted
children from our files shows (for further details see page 258) that
whereas 82.2 per cent were below normal in head size at the start of
treatment, *all but 37 of the children moved to an above-average rate
of growth* in head size over the fourteen-month period covered by
the survey, and in fact the average rate of growth during treatment
was 254 per cent of normal for that age.

We must consider also the fact that the visual maturation that is
occurring in the tiny brain-injured children who are reading exceeds
that of well children who cannot deal visually with the small print
as the hurt children do.

It must be remembered that visual maturation is a *brain* process
since the visual pathways, along with the auditory, tactile, olfactory
and gustatory pathways, actually make up virtually all of the back of
the central nervous system itself.

To say that one is maturing or growing the visual pathways is quite
literally to say that one is maturing or growing the brain.

To say that one is growing the auditory or tactile pathways is also
to say that one is growing the brain itself.

It must be remembered that many of the children who come to The
Institutes blind, end up reading. It must be remembered that many of
the children who come to The Institutes deaf, end up hearing and
talking. It must be remembered that many of the children who come
to The Institutes without feeling of any kind, end up able to distinguish between very small objects by feel alone.

These sensory pathways make up the back or sensory half of the
central nervous system.

As regards the motor pathways, it must be remembered that many children come to The Institutes completely paralyzed and end up walking. It must be remembered that many children come to The Institutes unable to move a finger, hand or arm and end up writing. It must be remembered that many children come to The Institutes unable to make a sound and end up talking.

These motor pathways make up the front or motor half of the central nervous system.

The motor and sensory pathways taken together with their interconnections *are* the brain.

I must hasten to add parenthetically that there are also children who come to The Institutes blind or deaf or insensate or paralyzed or speechless who remain so, and these children are our failures.

At any rate, these facts and others would tend to make us believe that in these children the brain can be made to grow just as the body can be made to grow since function determines structure in the brain as well as in the body.

There are tremendous amounts of evidence to support this view among the world's leading neurophysiologists. Two outstanding examples will illustrate this.

First, there is the work of that brilliant Russian neurosurgeon and neurophysiologist, the late Boris Klosovskii, who was Chief of Neurosurgery at the Academy of Medical Sciences of the USSR in Moscow.

So important do we believe Professor Klosovskii's work to be that both Carl Delacato and I traveled to Moscow to see it and to talk to Klosovskii.

Here is what he had done. He had taken newborn litters of kittens and puppies and had divided them into two exactly equal groups, one as the experimental group and the other as the control group. Into the experimental group he had placed a female kitten and into the control group he had placed a sister from the same litter. He then did the same thing with each of the male kittens from each litter and he divided the puppies in the same fashion until he had two perfectly matched groups, each containing kittens and puppies from each of the litters.

The kittens and puppies in the control group were then permitted to grow in the usual way in which kittens and puppies normally grow. The experimental animals, however, were simply placed on a slowly revolving turntable and lived there throughout the experiment.

The only difference, then, in what had happened to each of the groups was that the experimental group saw a *moving* world while the control group saw only as much as newborn kittens and puppies normally see.

When the animals were ten days old, Klosovskii began to sacrifice matched pairs of the kittens and puppies and to take their brains. He had sacrificed the last of them by the nineteenth day of life.

What Klosovskii found in the brains of his experimental animals should be required reading for every parent of a small child.

The experimental animals had from 22.8 to 35.0 per cent more growth in vestibular areas of the brain than did the control animals.

To state the same thing in clearer language, in ten to nineteen days of seeing a moving world, the experimental kittens and puppies had almost one third more brain growth in balance areas of the brain than did their brothers and sisters who had not seen a moving world.

This is the more astonishing when one considers that a ten-day-old kitten or puppy or even a nineteen-day-old kitten or puppy is not yet much of a creature; yet the animals that saw a moving world had actually almost one third more brain growth (and some of them more than one third more). Just what does more growth mean? Did Klosovskii see one third larger number of brain cells in his microscope? Not at all; he saw the same number of brain cells but one third larger and one third more mature.

When I consider the control animals, I think of average three- and four-year-old children, and when I think of the experimental kittens and puppies with one third more brain growth, I think of our hurt kids who are reading. Then I cannot help wondering what would have happened if Klosovskii had taken a third group of kittens and puppies and put them in darkness. Would they have had one third less brain growth and would they have reminded me of those little Xingu babies who live in dark huts?

But Klosovskii did not have a third group of animals, and thus we cannot know how it would have been.

Perhaps, however, we can conclude what might have happened had Klosovskii had a third group by going to the opposite end of the world to meet that genius David Krech, whose brilliant work at Berkeley supplies me with my second example.

Dr. Krech is not only a scientist whose impeccable conclusions are beyond question; he is more than that, perhaps much more than that, since in addition to great scientific knowledge he also has great wisdom. This is a wonderful combination because science is not always wise, nor is all wisdom always scientific. How I wish that gentle, witty David Krech could be heard by all parents rather than only by those who read scientific journals.

Dr. Krech has spent an important portion of his life repeating an experiment with slight modifications each time. He begins by raising two sets of infant rats. One set lives in an environment of sensory deprivation; that is to say, an environment in which there is little to see, hear or feel. The other rats are raised in an environment of sensory enrichment; that is to say, one in which there is a great deal to see and hear and feel.

He then tests the intelligence of the rats by such tests as putting food in mazes. The deprived rats either cannot find the food or find it with great difficulty. The rats raised in the enriched environment find the food easily and quickly.

He then sacrifices the rats and examines their brains.

"Rats which have been raised in sensory deprivation," he notes, "have small, stupid, undeveloped brains, while rats which have been raised in sensory enrichment have large, intelligent, highly developed brains."

He then states his scientific conclusion which, befitting a world-famous neurophysiologist, is scientifically immaculate.

"It would be scientifically unjustifiable," says Dr. Krech, "to conclude that because this is true in rats that it is also true in people."

Then he adds great wisdom.

"And it would be socially criminal to conclude that it is not true in people."

The last time I had the opportunity to see Dr. Krech I asked him if he envisioned doing anything about people.

His eyes twinkled as he replied, "I have not devoted my life to this for the purpose of creating more intelligent rats."

Amen.

David Krech has a problem. He cannot turn his rats into people and thus prove conclusively that human brains also grow by sensory stimulation.

We, too, have a problem. For years we have been giving human children sensory stimulation and seeing them progress, sometimes extraordinarily. However, we cannot make our children into rats and sacrifice them to examine their brains, although there are those who insist that we do.

I remember a good example of this many years ago.

I was having the privilege of addressing a group of graduate physicians at the Medical School of the University of São Paulo, Brazil.

Although Dr. Veras was with me, the dean of the Medical School was translating for me since my Portuguese did not extend very far beyond that necessary for good manners.

After the speech there were a good many highly intelligent questions and an extremely good-humored exchange of comments. There seems, however, to be one in almost every audience; the dean nodded to a man in the first row with his hand raised who turned out to be a neurologist.

He aroused my suspicions first by turning around to face the audience while he asked me his question. Then he spoke for twenty minutes. Now there are no twenty-minute questions. There are twenty-minute speeches, but no twenty-minute questions. As he continued to talk, some of the doctors began to mutter. *"Stupido,"* several of them were saying, and even with my limited Portuguese I could make out what that meant.

When at long last he had finished his question, the dean boiled down the twenty-minute harangue. "The doctor," the dean said, a little apologetically, "wants to know how you know a child is well if you succeed in making him well."

"Our standards are simple, sir. If a child acts in every way like other children his age, and if we can't tell him from his peers, and his parents can't, and if his doctor can't, and if his teacher can't, and if his playmates can't, we call that well."

There were friendly smiles around the room as the dean translated.

The doctor was not to be silenced by the dean or by his colleagues and again he turned his back and made another twenty-minute speech. This time there were less polite protests, and he was obviously being invited to sit down.

This time the dean was clearly embarrassed. "It is a ridiculous question," he said, "and there is no need to answer it. He wants to know if when you have successfully treated a child you then examine his brain physically to see if it is now well."

I responded to the dean's embarrassment. "If I may answer him in the same spirit in which he asked the question I'd be glad to."

The dean smiled and answered me with an Americanism, "Be my guest."

"In the United States we have some quaint customs and even some rigidly enforced taboos. One of them is that if we succeed in bringing a hurt child to total function, his parents don't want us to then operate on his brain to see what it looks like inside. It is also a tribal taboo, since even the government would be opposed to our doing so. I've noticed that these same customs seem to exist here in Brazil, too. However, the doctor does not seem to share these customs and concerns, so perhaps we could have a look at his own brain to see precisely what happens to it before and after treatment."

The dean smiled and translated, and on that cheery note the meeting broke up.

When people do not choose to be reasonable, they are not restrained by the bands of reason.

One of my great personal heroes, Dr. Jonas Salk, once said to me, "Now go on, don't stop to prove over and over again what you've already proven. The bright people will understand it the first time you say it. Those who don't want to understand, won't understand it if you say it five thousand times."

David Krech can't make his rats into people.

We can't make our children into rats.

I don't suppose we'll be able to actually watch human brains operate for a long time to come.

But there is a moment in history when the circumstantial evidence to support a view mounts to the point where to ignore the evidence and continue to do nothing while childrens' future lives are at stake becomes in every way as criminal as to introduce dangerous techniques without sufficient evidence to support them.

The brain, it would appear, grows through use exactly as a biceps does.

The problem in the brain-injured child is precisely that the brain injury acts as a barrier to the reception of incoming sensory stimulation over the visual, auditory and tactile pathways, just as it may act as a barrier to outgoing motor response.

How to penetrate this barrier. This was the question on which all treatment of the brain-injured child must rest.

How do you get a stimulus into the brain through a barrier? Again I can hear so clearly the words of my neurology professor thirty years ago.

"There are three ways of insuring the transmission of central nervous system stimuli. You must increase the stimuli in frequency, intensity and duration."

Frequency, Intensity, Duration.

These three words become the most important words in the life of the brain-injured child--along with two others, family and love. Taken together, these five words are the five that offer a brain-injured child a chance to become a first-class, functioning human being. Family and love are well understood in relation to children. Frequency, intensity and duration are far less understood. What do they mean?

If a message sent to the brain through visual, auditory or tactile pathways does not arrive either because it was not strong enough or because a barrier in the form of a brain injury exists (or for any other reason), there are three ways to help the message get through; namely an increase in its frequency, intensity or duration.

Let's suppose that a pressure on the skin of the arm is the message we wish to transmit to the brain. We have gently squeezed the arm and the message is not received. As an example, we might have my wife squeezing my arm to let me know that it is time to go home so that our hosts can go to bed. But I am deeply involved in a conversation with another guest. She squeezes my arm gently but the message does not arrive and I do not notice. Being a first-class rehabilitationist, she knows precisely how to reach my brain. (I must admit that as a wife she *always* seems to have known it.)

First she tries increasing the frequency of the stimulus. Instead of squeezing my arm every five minutes, she squeezes it ten times in a row. She knows that frequency facilitates transmission.

If that doesn't work, she tries increasing the duration. She doesn't only squeeze my arm but she keeps it squeezed. She knows that duration facilitates transmission of tactile messages to the brain.

If that doesn't work, she resorts to the last way to facilitate transmission to the brain. She increases the stimulus in intensity. Instead of squeezing my arm, she pinches my arm, and she pinches harder and harder until, however deeply I am engaged in conversation, I get the message.

"Do you think we should be going, dear?"

She smiles sweetly.

I have an idea that other wives who aren't even experts on neurophysiology know this instinctively.

If you are perhaps saying to yourself that of course it would work on you or on me because we aren't brain-injured, I would urge you to wait until you've read the chapter concerning who is brain-injured and who isn't. Then decide how firm a stand you can safely take on whether you or I aren't brain-injured.

However, because you haven't yet read that chapter, let's take a look at how frequency, intensity and duration facilitate brain transmission in an auditory sense in a human being very clearly brain-injured.

Not long ago we were having dinner with some friends whose father is ninety years old and who remains active and intelligent. He is, however, paying the price of advancing age. The death of cells in his auditory pathways is preceding the death of cells in other areas of the brain.

Grandfather had enjoyed a cocktail with us in the living room.

"Is everybody ready for dinner?" said our hostess.

"Ready for what?" asked her father.

"Ready for dinner, ready for dinner," repeated his daughter (frequency).

"What?" shouted her father.

"Dinner, dinner, dinner, dinner, dinner," said the daughter smiling (duration).

"What did you say?" yelled her father.

"DINNER," screamed his daughter (intensity).

"Stop yelling at me and let's go eat," said the old man with great dignity.

Let's consider visual facilitation with a child who is so severely brain-injured at six years of age that he is unable to distinguish outlines and has only the light reflex of a newborn infant, which is to say that from a functional standpoint he is totally blind and does not even bother to keep his eyes open.

Here again we will use frequency, intensity and duration to ensure that the visual message of light actually reaches his brain.

We open his eyes with our fingers and flash light in his eyes as many as one hundred times in five minutes (frequency).

We use a strong light (intensity).

We continue to do so for many weeks if it is necessary (duration).

So frequency, intensity and duration are words that have overwhelming importance in the homes of all children on the program of The Institutes.

Although all three of these words have the greatest importance for all children, there are varying times in some childrens' lives when one or another of these words is of overwhelming importance.

An excellent example of this is the brain-injured child who is in a profound coma. This state is as near the state of actual death as it is possible for a human being to get. A very large number of human beings in a profound coma do, in fact, die.

Coma frequently follows a severe brain injury; after the injury, the brain is swollen in a state which is called edema which in itself tends to produce coma. In the days following the injury, that swelling tends to reduce and, as it does, many children regain total consciousness. However, all brain edema should be gone at the end of thirty to sixty days. Certainly by ninety days this swelling should be over and the child should have regained consciousness.

Unfortunate indeed has been the child who has not by then regained consciousness, since the chances are high that he will now, sooner or later, slip across that line from deathlike coma to death itself.

We have seen children who have been in coma for six months or a year or two years or four years. A number of years ago I was asked by the Brazilian Government to see a girl who had been in coma for eighteen years. At eight years old she had been hit by a bus and now she was twenty-six years old.

There are two ways that we can deal with a child in coma following a brain injury. We can either patiently maintain him until he one day crosses that line, or we can give him a highly organized and carefully planned program of neurological organization aimed at reaching his brain through the frequency, intensity and duration with which we put visual, auditory and tactile stimulation into his brain.

At The Institutes we have employed the highly organized approach for brain-injured children for more than ten years. We now employ a coma kit and a coma team of physician, a nurse, and a therapist to carry out this program. We put visual, auditory, tactile and even olfactory and gustatory stimulation into the child's brain for hours on end using frequency, intensity and duration.

These three.

But the greatest of these is intensity.

At least for the child in coma.

We shine into his eyes a powerful light.

In his ears we make a huge noise.

We pinch his skin mightily.

We put aromatic spirits of ammonia under his nose.

We put a pinch of horse-radish on his tongue.

For with this child we require tremendous intensity, over all else, to penetrate the barrier of brain injury which has made him functionally blind, functionally deaf and functionally insensate, for that is precisely what coma is!

Through every pathway that goes into his brain we are pounding in a message, and that message is:

Child, you are not allowed to resign from the human race. Come back! Come back! Come back!

I wish I could report that every time our coma team has engaged in our coma program the child has promptly come back. That would not be true.

But more than 50 per cent of the children in a state of coma on whom we have worked have come back, and generally quickly, although in no case had they been in a coma less than sixty days and in several cases it had been years.

In coma, frequency, intensity and duration are all of staggering importance. But the most important is intensity.

To a highly alert but paralyzed and speechless brain-injured child, frequency, intensity and duration are all of great importance, but the most important is frequency.

To a conscious but extensively brain-injured child, frequency, intensity and duration are all of great importance, but the most important of these is duration.

It is in these three ways that we penetrate the barrier of brain injury.

I can best conclude this chapter as to what is going on in the brain by summarizing in a single paragraph all we have learned about the human brain and then summarizing all we do at The Institutes in another single paragraph.

Here in essence is what we have learned.

The world has regarded brain growth and development as if it were predetermined and unalterable. Instead, brain growth and development is a dynamic and ever-changing process. It is a process that can be stopped (as it is by severe brain injury). This is a process that can be slowed (as it is by moderate brain injury), but, most significantly, it is a process that can be speeded (and were it not so, the far-behind brain-injured child could never catch up).

It is a paragraph that says a great deal. It is a paragraph that is easily proven by the simple comparison of a severely brain-injured child's neurological age (let's say 2 months) with his chronological age (let's say 130 months). For this child, brain growth and development have stopped at 2 months but time has continued for 130 months.

It is proven by the comparison of a moderately brain-injured child's neurological age (let's say 24 months) with his chronological age (let's say 48 months). For this child brain growth and development have slowed to exactly half of normal.

The final sentence is proven by the severely brain-injured child (neurological age 2 months—chronological age 130 months) who now begins a program of neurological organization. A year later he has a neurological age of 26 months and a chronological age of 142 months. In one year of elapsed time he has grown two years' worth. For him the process has been speeded.

The remaining paragraph is the one that tells all we do at The Institutes.

In recognition of the fact that function determines structure, and that in order for function to take place in a brain-injured child, we must facilitate the transmission of brain messages by increasing the stimuli, therefore:

All we do at The Institutes for the Achievement of Human Potential is to give a child visual, auditory and tactile stimulation with increased frequency, intensity and duration as well as unlimited opportunity to function in full recognition of the orderly way in which the brain grows.

That, as I have said, is all we do. It is fair to add that in doing so we employ five principles, dozens of methods and hundreds of techniques. Nonetheless, they all fit into the above paragraph.

This chapter explains what at this moment in history we believe is probably going on in the brain and is probably the explanation for the results we are presently achieving with brain-injured children.

Perhaps on one future day, in light of whatever advances have been made by then, we shall believe a different thing to be the reason for what is happening.

But today all of this seems to us in Philadelphia to be the most reasonable and logical possibility.

23.

THE DEATH OF TEMPLE FAY

It had been six years since Dr. Fay had left The Institutes, and I had missed him very much. I had seen him only once since then. That had been in 1960 when I had met him unexpectedly in an international meeting in Detroit where we were both speakers. He had been extremely cordial and kindly and had charmed me as easily as ever.

But I had not seen him since and now it was 1963 and I found myself worrying about him with increasing frequency. I had heard rumors that he was not well and I dreaded that I might one day waken to read in a headline that Fay was dead. Despite our separation I still considered him in every way my mentor and preceptor and I his devoted student and disciple.

When the news came, it was worse than I wanted and not as bad as I feared. Fay was not dead but he had had a stroke.

Bob and I had a talk. I wanted to go immediately to Fay and offer him the full facilities of The Institutes. If anyone in the world deserved the best treatment available for strokes, it was Temple Fay who had contributed so much to the knowledge of what to do about them.

Bob went immediately to see Dr. Fay and offer him the full facilities of The Institutes.

While Bob was gone, I sat in my office and thought. What in the world would that giant of a man with the towering intellect do with a stroke? Would he be paralyzed and speechless, and if he was, could he possibly exist in that way or would he die of sheer agonized frustration?

I remember how often Temple Fay had stepped to a blackboard and, with skilled ease, drawn a brain in profile and said, "Right precisely here is where his lesion must be," as he discussed some brain-injured person.

He would mark the spot with an X. So great was his love of the human brain that he was unable to discuss it without obvious relish.

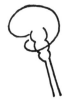

FIGURE 22

Many who listened to him mistook his delight in the human brain for delight in brain injury and considered him cruel and inhuman when he drew the brain and placed his X to locate the pathology.

Three hours later my brother returned and his face wore a happy grin which relieved me vastly.

Bob couldn't help giggling as he told me his story. Fay, despite a severe stroke, hadn't changed a bit.

After greeting Bob, the first thing Fay had done was to take a large piece of paper; on it, with easy skill, he had drawn a human brain in profile.

"Now my lesion," Fay had said to Bob with great relish, "has to be precisely here," making an X.

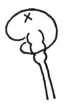

FIGURE 23

Bob had brought the paper back with him since Fay had been sure I would want to see it. As I said earlier, Fay could no more resist teaching than he could resist breathing, and his brain, like everybody else's, was teaching material.

Fay, Bob reported, had been partially paralyzed initially but had been unwilling to put up with that for more than a few weeks. He had, in fact, only one remaining problem. Fay had a transcortical aphasia.

Transcortical aphasia is perhaps the lightest of all speech problems, but it is perhaps the most frustrating of all speech problems.

The patient with transcortical aphasia has no problem in speaking and can, in fact, speak easily and fluently and accurately—except for one little thing. He cannot manage the specific names of people or things. This can be maddening.

If you hold up a pencil and say to a person with transcortical aphasia, "What is this?" it is quite likely that he'll respond something like this:

"Oh, that's a . . . You know what it is, it's a . . . You know, you write with it . . . What the devil do you call it . . . It's not a pen, it's a . . . You know, it has lead and it's wood . . ."

If you then hold up a pen and say, "What's this?" it is quite possible that he'll say:

"Oh, of course, it's not a pencil . . . It's . . . You know, ink . . . It's Waterman's, Schaeffer's . . . You know, you write with it."

If the reader is presently feeling a mild discomfort, then I hasten to point out that all normal people experience this exact same thing for brief periods of time.

Have you ever walked down the street with your mother and met your best friend and had trouble introducing them? "I'd like you to meet . . . that is, she is . . . ah, she's . . ."

Well, she's your mother, that's who she is, but just for the moment it escapes you. You know how awful it is. Well that's how it is with the transcortical aphasic all the time.

And Fay had transcortical aphasia.

Bob offered Fay all the facilities of The Institutes to use as he wished for as long as he wished.

It was then that we saw Fay at his most magnificent.

Speaking carefully and groping for the words he wanted to use, and coping with the staggering frustration of having a transcortical aphasia, Fay said what only Fay in all the world could say.

Fay had told Bob to thank us for our kind offer and to say he found himself with a little spare time. He told Bob to tell me that if I would send the chief of the Speech Pathology Department down to his house every day, *he would be glad to teach her about transcortical aphasia.* I laughed until my sides hurt and so did Bob. I stopped worrying about Temple Fay.

A few months thereafter The International Forum for Rehabilitation voted to give its highest honor, the Statuette With Pedestal, to Temple Fay. I was deeply honored to be asked to make the presentation at the Annual Dinner. I also was chosen to put the bell on the cat. I had to be sure he attended the meeting, which is an extremely elegant affair and which was to be held that year in the stately Lincoln Room of the Union League.

The meeting was only two weeks off when I decided I could delay no longer. Since the recipient is never announced in advance, I decided to enlist Mrs. Fay's help.

I called her during the day and found her beside herself. Dr. Fay was in the hospital, gravely ill with an extremely dangerous chest condition in addition to his stroke. He could have no visitors, and it seemed clear they did not believe he would survive. I mumbled my sympathy, explained the situation and, extremely ill at ease, I asked Mrs. Fay if she might put in an appearance and accept the award for Dr. Fay if his condition permitted her to do so. Mrs. Fay's attention was obviously distracted and she proposed that I call back the following week.

I was disconsolate since it did not seem that Fay would survive long enough to receive the honor which I was sure he would truly treasure. How unfair and ironic it seemed to me that this heroic man, who had been the target of a thousand invidious attacks by lesser men, should die without even knowing of this major tribute.

With heavy heart I phoned Mrs. Fay the following Monday, just five days before the presentation.

When Mrs. Fay answered the phone she was talking in a very subdued voice and I immediately feared the worst, but the worst had not happened. There was a different reason altogether for her quietness.

As I asked her if she could come to the dinner, I heard the click of someone picking up an extension and a tiny, tiny voice, but nonetheless Fay's voice, said, "Glenn, now just what is that all about?"

Fay had decided not to die for a while yet, probably out of precisely the same curiosity that had caused him to be willing to see me that very first day in his office almost a quarter of a century earlier.

It was obvious that Mrs. Fay had told him about the award.

His voice was so tiny I could barely hear him and he still had some trace of his transcortical aphasia. It was obvious that he was having great trouble breathing.

He obviously wanted to hear me tell him about the award, and so I explained it to him again. I ended up by saying that I knew he had been ill and wasn't quite himself yet, but that if he could spare Mrs. Fay just long enough for us to make the presentation to her, we would send a car for her and have her driven right back home again.

It was not what Fay had in mind.

I strained to hear.

"Will it be black tie?" asked Fay.

I could hardly believe my ears. I told him it would be.

Could he come in a wheel chair? asked the faint voice.

Of course he could.

Could he bring his oxygen?

Of course he could.

Could he bring an attendant, asked the voice I could barely hear.

Of course, and we would send a car for him and Mrs. Fay and his daughter, Marion. They could arrive any time they pleased and we would stop wherever we were in the dinner and make the presentation and he could then leave immediately.

His voice was just a little stronger when he asked me the final question.

"How long," he inquired, "do you think I should make my speech?"

After I hung up, I sat and looked at the telephone for a long time.

Fay was late for the dinner and I remember looking at the candlelight reflecting off the elegant silverware and the burnished paneled walls of the Lincoln Room and praying that he had survived and would survive this night.

Then the great paneled doors, twice as high as a man, opened and there was Fay, faultlessly attired in his tuxedo, sitting in his wheel chair as if it were the throne of old Rome itself and he, the Emperor. With Mrs. Fay on one side of his chair and Marion on the other, he swept into the room.

Every person in the room rose to his feet and found himself applauding as Dr. Fay, with wheel chair, oxygen tank and attendant, was rolled into place beside my chair.

"Never before," said Fay in my ear, "has there been so funereal an entrance into this august body."

I dared to disagree. "I believe, sir, it is much more like Louis Pasteur coming before the French Academy."

We finished dinner, although Fay barely touched his food. His conversation was cheerful and he asked the name of every person in the room he didn't know personally.

I presented the Statuette.

Fay made his speech from his wheel chair in a voice that could barely be heard across the room, stopping frequently to take oxygen.

He spoke for thirty-five minutes, and there was not a sound except that tiny voice filling that great room.

He allowed himself just five minutes to cover all of past glory. He spoke briefly of his discovery of human refrigeration saying neither how he had been attacked for it nor that it was now used in every modern hospital in the world. Five minutes altogether.

Then for thirty minutes he talked about tomorrow and what must yet be done, and what he said was prophetic. He spoke much of us at The Institutes and he spoke of us with respect and with deep affection and with humor.

Fay was in every sense a physician, and Fay knew that his moments were numbered, but this he did not say. But I knew that he knew, and he knew that I knew. In that thirty-five minutes, with joy and with happiness and with humor, he passed the torch.

He also handed us a rich heritage both publicly and privately. That night will live in my heart and mind as long as I live. There was not a soul present who did not know that this was the most momentous of evenings.

The party lasted until after midnight and Fay was the last one out the door except for John Tini who was pushing his wheel chair.

I was afraid to call Mrs. Fay the following morning for fear the excitement had been too much for Dr. Fay.

"He hasn't looked so well in years." Mrs. Fay reported. "He told me to ask you if the press was there last night."

Fay operated on Fay's terms.

A few weeks later it suited Dr. Temple Fay to die, and so he did.

When he died most people thought he was a hundred years old. This was because they had known him to be a famous professor thirty years earlier and assumed he had been seventy then. But in truth he had been thirty-eight then.

Fay was sixty-eight when he died.

"The first condition for immortality is death."

By 1963 Dr. Temple Fay had met *all* the conditions for immortality.

24.

PARENTS ARE NOT THE PROBLEM: PARENTS ARE THE ANSWER

When we human beings get a myth firmly planted in our minds, it becomes almost impossible to get it out. Such a myth can make us know what we're going to see before we see it. Then, no matter what actually happens, we see what we *thought* we were going to see.

To put it differently, so much of what we "see" doesn't start with the image sent by the eye to the brain, as it should, but starts instead within the brain. In the same way, so much of what we "hear" isn't what was sent by our ears to our brain, but is instead what we expected to hear.

Professional people are by no means immune to such myths, and the greatest of all these professional myths is the one that maintains that, if it weren't for parents, everything would be absolutely great in the world of children.

This myth so dearly loved by educators, special educators, psychologists, librarians, pediatricians, therapists and a host of others who deal with parents and children, just isn't so.

Parents are not the problem: Parents are the answer! The greater the number of problems a child has, and the more serious the problems, the more important this basic fact becomes.

Parents are not the problem with children: Parents are the answer.

I see this with crystal clarity at The Institutes in relation to fathers, whom I take as an example because I am a male.

During the intensive week which both parents and child spend with us at The Institutes (and which I described briefly in the very beginning of this book), we teach every father to do a complex program for his child and we make him *reasonably* competent. He will never do the program as competently as I do it for the simple reason that in all his life he will never do the program one tenth as much as I've done it.

But that doesn't mean that I can treat his daughter Mary better than he can. He is her father and I am not. The combination of being reasonably competent *and* her father (which he is) is much more powerful than being highly competent and *not* her father (which I am not). I can make him reasonably competent, but he can't make me her father, even a little bit.

What is true of her father is even more true of her mother.

And oh, what myths there are about mothers. Oh, what sly innuendos and what outright lies, and what outrageous ones. The myths about mothers are so outrageous that they would be absolutely hilarious—if the consequences weren't so tragic and disastrous.

The unspoken law holds that all mothers are idiots and they have no truth in them. The tragic consequence of this is that almost no professional people talk to mothers, and God knows that almost nobody listens to them. What makes this so especially sad is that mothers know more about their own children than anyone else in the world.

The myth says that the trouble with mothers is that they are too emotionally involved with their children. Now surely that suggests that somehow things would be better if mothers were *not* emotionally involved with their children. Have you ever thought what the world would be like if mothers were not emotionally involved with their children?

Every time I think of that, it occurs to me that I'm sure mother alligators are less emotionally involved with baby alligators than mother people are with baby people. But I wonder if that's better for the baby alligators. Or is that maybe why they are baby alligators instead of baby people, because their mothers are not emotionally involved with them? The myth goes on to say that *because* mothers are emotionally involved with their children, they can't be objective about them. I suppose if a mother has got a well kid she can afford her little myth that this kid is going to be President or the first lady pope or whatever. Why not? I suppose somebody is going to be, and who's got a right to deny that this may be the one? If a mother has got a hurt kid, she can't afford any myths, and nobody in the world knows it better than mother does. Nobody in all of the world. But professionals insist that mothers don't want to know if the children are hurt.

Let me tell you a story. Again, this would be highly amusing if it weren't so tragic. In every hospital in the world, the instant a child is born, a struggle begins between the staff and the mother, with the mother making every effort to get her baby and the staff making every effort to prevent her from getting her baby. All mother wants is to get her hands on the baby, get the staff out of the room, strip the baby down to the buff and start counting. Five toes on this foot, five toes on this foot, two eyes, two ears, one nose. Now if mother doesn't want to know, what the devil is the inventory for? Why has she taken it if the truth is that she doesn't want to know? When we get smarter, the first thing we'll do when a baby is born is give it to the mommy and say, "Here's a check sheet. Please check off whether he's got everything or not." Did any reader who is a mother fail to take an inventory of her child as early as possible? Well now, if you didn't want to know whether something was wrong, why were you counting?

Now consider the next step. The Institutes for the Achievement of Human Potential have the most sophisticated records of brain-injured children in the world, the largest number of brain-injured children that were ever treated by a single system in history. Those records are very thorough. In the histories we take from the parents, among the hundreds of questions we ask are these three: (A) Who first decided this child had a problem, (B) When? (C) Why? If you go into our record room and take out a thousand charts and look up that question, in more than nine hundred out of a thousand charts it was *mother* who first decided the child had a problem, and generally she had a *hell* of a time convincing anybody else.

Here's a typical case history of a severely brain-injured child, who was severely brain-injured from birth. (By the way, if it's a moderately brain-injured child, same story; it just takes longer—3 years. If it's mildly brain-injured, it takes still longer—six years. Same story always.)

At three months of age, Mother says, "Doctor, there's something wrong with my baby." And the doctor says, *"All* mothers think that." At six months of age, Mother says, "Doctor, there's something *wrong* with my baby." And he says, "Don't compare one baby to another; they're all different from each other." At nine months of age, Mother's voice is going up. It has a slight edge of hysteria, not because she *knows* she's got a hurt child, but because nobody will listen to her. And she says, "Doctor, there's something wrong with my baby!" And he says, "He's a little slow, but he'll grow out of it." At eighteen months of age, Mother says (she's very calm now, she's made up her mind), "Doctor, are *you* going to do something about my baby or am I going to get another doctor?" And that's the day the doctor discovers severely brain-injured children. That very day. And then an astonishing thing happens. He says, "Not only is something wrong with your baby, but he's hopeless."

Now the question is, what changed that day? Did the baby actually go from being totally normal to totally hopeless in one day? Did Mother change? That's what she's been saying all along. Only one thing changed that day—the professional mind. And then these emotionally involved, fool mothers say an interesting thing; they say, "Doctor, for eighteen months I've been telling you something was wrong and you've been saying it wasn't, and you were wrong. Now you're saying he's hopeless—and you're wrong again."

The myth goes on to say that the problem with mothers is that they're not objective about their children, that they're unrealistic. And then it goes on to describe this unrealistic mother. I have learned that mothers of brain-injured children are so realistic they scare me. They've been laughed at by professionals so long that they're afraid to say anything hopeful about the child for fear they'll be laughed at again, and the consequence of that is that every once in a while I see a little three-year-old kid and I say, "Does he understand the word 'Mommy'?" And Mother says, "Well now I can't prove it . . ." and I say, "Now look, Mom, he's not taking college board entrance requirements, I just want to know if you think he understands 'Mommy' or not." There's nobody more realistic than mothers of brain-injured children.

That unrealistic mother—I do see her every once in a while. It isn't that she doesn't exist, she exists all right. And when I see her she's exactly as painted. She brings in a little three-year-old lump and puts him on my floor. He can't move, he can't make sounds and she tells me about how he can walk and talk. And I have found my unrealistic mother. The only thing is, I've been led to believe that she's unrealistic *because* she's got a brain-injured child. When I find this gal—she's unrealistic about *everything*. She's simply an unrealistic human being who happens to be the mother of a brain-injured child.

I mean, there's nothing about being unrealistic that keeps you from being pregnant, is there? Indeed, there may be some things about being unrealistic that lead to pregnancy. It's quite possible for unrealistic people to become mothers and so, when I find her, she's just exactly as painted. What is lied about is not what she's like; it's her frequency. Because I'm told she's everybody. And I see her regularly . . . every three years. She's one in a thousand mothers.

As I said earlier: *Parents are not the problem with children: Parents are the answer.*

All over the world today, a sad, sad drama is being acted out. All over the world parents are taking their brain-injured children to institutions for what is solemnly called "Evaluation and Diagnosis."

Such evaluations are generally extremely expensive and require the child to be an inpatient for ten days or two weeks. At the end of this period of time it is quite possible for the parents (if they are unlucky) to get back the child and a large bill without anybody even saying good-by to them. This approach suggests that children exist for the purpose of being evaluated. It is a quaint view of life.

If the parents are luckier, at the end of the child's hospitalization, in addition to receiving the child and the large bill, somebody says good-by to them, which generally means that someone sits down with them and explains that they have done this test and this test and this test. The conversation then goes like this:

PARENTS: "Yes?"

PRO: "As a consequence of all these tests we have diagnosed your child as 'Severely Mentally Retarded.' "

PARENTS: "Yes?"

PRO: "Well that's it. Your child is severely mentally retarded."

PARENTS: "But what does that *mean?*"

PRO: "Why that means your son can't *do* what other children his age can do."

DAD: (After long silence) "You're pulling my leg. You have to be. You wouldn't dare bring my child in here and keep him ten days and do painful things to him and then give us a large bill and *dare* to tell us that he can't do the things that other kids his age can do. Why that's exactly what *we* told *you* when we brought him here. We don't need to pay anybody to tell us what he can't do. His mother here is the world's leading authority on what he can't do—and what he can do. That's all we've talked about every night for the last four years. You're joking, and it's a damned bad joke."

PRO: "No, I'm not joking. I've been in this field for five years and I'm telling you your son is severely mentally retarded and you better face up to it."

PARENT: "We didn't bring our son here to be told what he can't do, and we didn't bring him here to have you put a name on not being able to do what other kids his age do.

"We brought him here to find out two things. First: *Why* he can't do what other kids do, and Second: What we're going to *do* about it. If you can't tell us the answer to these questions, we'll look until we find somebody who can."

And, as usual with parents, they are the two exactly proper questions that must be answered if we're going to solve the problems of brain-injured children.

As I think I mentioned before,

Parents are not the problem with children: Parents are the answer.

It took me a very long time to learn this in the face of all the myths I lived with, but I finally learned it.

Most people think that the reason we teach parents to program their children instead of doing it ourselves is because it is so much cheaper for parents.

Certainly it is true that it would cost huge sums of money if we were going to actually treat the kids seven days a week for eight, ten or twelve hours a day as the parents do. But that's not why we have the parents treat the children.

The reason is that we know without question that if parents are taught thoroughly what is going on and why we do what we do and precisely how to do it, then the simple fact is that parents can do it *better* than we can do it. *Better* than Glenn Doman. *Better* than Hazel Doman. *Better* than Gretchen Kerr. *Better* than Elaine Lee. *Better* than Roselise Wilkinson. *Better* than Suzy Aisen. *Better* than Ann Ball.

The reason that parents can treat kids better than we can, if they know what they're doing, is very simple.

Much as everyone on the staff loves brain-injured children, and love them they do, each individual kid is loved even more by his individual parents.

Parents are not the problem with brain-injured children: Parents are the answer.

25.

ON MOTIVATION

It's surprising, really, how few mothers ask me about motivation when you consider how much everybody else talks about it.

I suppose the reason why my particular mothers rarely ask me about motivation is that they are already experienced; being the mothers of brain-injured children who are sometimes so severely injured that they must be encouraged to breathe, my mothers are among the world's leading experts on motivating children.

Not being a mother of a brain-injured child, nor even a female, I was not equipped by nature to understand motivation instinctively, nor were the professionals who were my teachers able to enlighten me. I learned about motivation by experience, observation and thought. Not being able to handle it by instinct, it was necessary for me to define it in words. It is frequently advantageous to be able to put words to instinctive reactions. I am now able to talk about motivation and dare to do so to some of the best motivating mothers in the whole world. Frequently, the mothers who are the best instinctive motivators are the most grateful for being able to evaluate their own actions in words.

When on occasion one of my mothers does raise the question of motivation, she almost invariably puts the question properly: "How," she asks, "can I motivate my child?" The very way she asks the question indicates that she knows the most important part of the answer. She does not ask why her child wasn't born motivated. Her question makes it clear that she believes that the problem of motivation lies within herself rather than being inborn with the child. She already knows the big secret.

For too long we have considered motivation to be a moral value, and an inherited moral value at that. This makes for convenient, quick analysis of a host of problems. If motivation is a product of morality and morality is inbred, then one can quickly understand how it is that highly motivated, highly competitive suburbanite achievers beget highly motivated, highly competitive, young suburbanite achievers with an occasional unmotivated underachiever exception to prove the rule. It also explains why the unmotivated, unemployed, crime-prone ghetto dwellers tend to beget the next generation of unmotivated, unemployed, crime-prone ghetto dwellers to swell the relief rolls, with an occasional highly motivated achiever exception to prove the rule.

Thus, we are shown how morality begets morality, motivation begets motivation and achievement begets achievement. Thus, we are shown how immorality reproduces immorality, lack of motivation reproduces lack of motivation and crime reproduces crime. Thus, drunken, poverty-stricken Navajos reproduce drunken, poverty-stricken Navajos; ignorant Australian aborigines reproduce ignorant Australian aborigines; starving Kalahari Bushmen reproduce starving Kalahari Bushmen; and so it goes.

Motivation is familial and inbred. It's a convenient thought. It's an easy thought. It would explain a lot. The only problem for me is that I don't believe it. I've lived in too many huts in too many jungles and too many deserts to believe it. It conflicts with all I see. It conflicts with all I know. It conflicts, I think, with the facts.

It is *not* that motivation begets success and that *lack* of motivation begets failure. It is quite the other way round. Success *creates* motivation. Failure *destroys* motivation.

There are a couple of similar words which have much to do with motivation. The words are *reward* and *punishment*. Success leads to reward which leads to motivation. Failure leads to punishment which leads to lack of motivation.

I have watched the fascinating process by which the brain-injured child pounds his way to function as a trout beats his way up impossible waterfalls against enormous odds. For more than a quarter century I have been a privileged observer of the brain-injured child trying to crawl across a room on his belly, moving against paralysis, against uncontrollable and unwanted movements, with incomplete vision, incomplete hearing, incomplete sensation, using his fingernails, his toenails, his teeth, using even the uncontrolled and unwanted movement if this chaotic flopping happens to push him forward and struggling onward against it when it pushes him backward.

Although I have watched this Olympian struggle on the part of a tiny child thousands of times, I remain forever involved as I sit silently watching. My knuckles whiten, my nails dig deep into my palms, I bite my lip, I am drenched in perspiration, I strain forward in my chair trying to push this heroic little child forward by my will if not by my prayer. Ten minutes pass and the struggle to crawl twenty feet continues and the tension increases as the child, against overwhelming odds, approaches the wall which is his goal. In my heart I cheer for him. I am not religious, but I pray for him. By God, I ask myself, why does he continue to try to gain so little at such cost in superhuman effort? But, by God, how I do admire this endlessly determined little bundle of terribly hurt humanity.

His hand flies out and touches the wall and the room explodes in wild applause. My office is filled with joy; parents, graduate students, physicians, staff are on their feet applauding, laughing, congratulating, and I find my own eyes wet with emotion for this little child. Not for a moment do I feel pity, which is a cheap and plentiful emotion; it is admiration which moves me to tears and, more than that, it is respect which courses down my cheek. No ballerina, no concert pianist, no Shakespearean actor in all of history ever received a more spontaneous or sincere ovation than this little bundle of hurt humanity now receives—and deserves.

I have, as I have said, experienced this drama thousands of times, and today I feel it not less but more than the first time I beheld this miracle of sorts, more than a quarter century ago. I suppose I *appreciate* it more.

I have been privileged to behold miracles of motivation, and I have watched those superb motivators, the mothers, countless times. And I have learned much.

I have learned that such monumental motivation has simple enough beginnings, simple not only in the children but in me, for in many ways I am childlike.

Motivation begins, clearly, with those ancient movers *punishment* and *reward*.

Punishment is so hard for the brain-injured child to comprehend that it certainly isn't the answer.

He can do so little that punishing him for a sin of commission is almost impossible. This leaves punishing him for a sin of omission as the only way to teach him the ancient law. Shall we punish him for not walking, not crawling, not creeping? Shall we punish him for not talking? Shall we punish him for not being able to do these things when in fact the only one in the world who is clearly not guilty for his inability is he?

If we cannot punish him for the transgressions he is unable to commit and if we cannot punish him for what he cannot do, how then shall he learn the ancient law of punishment?

If it is fear of punishment that prevents the child and me from doing those things we should *not* do, it is surely reward that causes the child and me to do the things we should do.

Again, it is easier for me to learn than it is for the child. As I work with my parents, my kids, my team members and my students, I am a much rewarded man. When I am wise enough and knowledgeable enough to design an individual program that brings about walking, talking, reading and writing in a child who was motionless, speechless or blind, I am rewarded far more than just being paid a salary. There are few rewards to compare. And when I am so rewarded, I am inspired to even greater efforts so that I may be so rewarded soon again and more often.

But what of the brain-injured child? What can he do to earn his reward? He is paralyzed and speechless and can neither do nor say the things that will earn his true reward. If this is so, how can we sincerely reward him? Should we then reward him for no accomplishment at all? To do so would be to teach him that in this hard world one is rewarded for nothing at all. To do so would be teaching him a lie. This would be understandable but very unwise.

It becomes clear that it is more difficult to teach a brain-injured child about punishment or reward than it is to teach a well child, and so where are we left?

Let's move back a bit to those predecessors of punishment and reward—*success* and *failure*.

Again let's consider me, for I am in most ways an uncomplicated person and childlike. Strange fellow that I am (as compared with you), I find myself with an extremely clear-cut view about success and failure. I find myself carefully avoiding doing those things at which I fail and repeating over and over again those things which I do well.

I *know* I should not. I *know* I should work hard at those things at which I fail so as to accomplish them and to avoid spending time at those things at which I invariably succeed since I am already accomplished at them. I *know* I would be a better person and that I would become more rounded if I did it the other way around.

Still, it occurs to me that I am round enough, and so I continue to avoid those things at which I fail and to return again and again to those things at which I succeed. I am sure that you do not behave in such an *undetermined* way. But I do.

I have never learned to play tennis nor can I carry a tune, and, despite all the insistence of my friends who play tennis beautifully or who sing superbly that I could easily learn, no one in the last forty years has succeeded in getting me onto a tennis court or to sing publicly since Miss Jeffries, my first grade teacher, blew her pitch pipe to give us *do* and then looked pained—and in my direction. I know I could learn if I wanted to. I just don't want to. I note with interest that all my friends who want to get me onto a tennis court play tennis beautifully and those who would head me for the concert stage sing beautifully.

I continue to avoid the things at which I fail. It's a weakness which I intend to keep.

On the other hand there are some things I do well and a few things that I do extremely well, and I know it. Try as I may to avoid it, I find myself doing those things over and over and over again. It goes like this. I do whatever it is that I do well. Since I *know* I do it well, I do it completely and confidently. It is almost always a pleasure to see something done well, and so when I am done you say, "Golly, but you did that well."

"Yes, I did do that rather well, didn't I?" I say. "Would you like to see me do that again?"

And so it goes.

In my weakness I am just like the kids whether they are overtly brain-injured or whether they are not. They also tend to avoid that at which they fail while repeating over and over again that at which they succeed.

By the very nature of the severely brain-injured child's brain injury, he is a born loser. He can frequently do absolutely nothing except breathe, and he almost always does that rather badly. Failure is the story of his life until help comes.

Now let us suppose that for some reason it would be a good idea to have a little brain-injured girl wrap her hands around a ¾″ bar and hang feet down supporting her weight from her hands. (This is, in fact, a first-rate idea for brain-injured children of all sizes and shapes and is a highly sophisticated idea which the staff of The Institutes for the Achievement of Human Potential in Philadelphia spent many years developing). Suppose, in fact, that your child, a four-year-old, let's say, is a patient at The Institutes in Philadelphia and that we have instructed you on the importance of her learning to hang by her hands for one minute even though she is unable to move and unable to speak.

Being a first-rate set of parents, you are most anxious to give your tiny paralyzed daughter every opportunity to be a whole functioning human being. Indeed, you would give anything in the world to bring that about.

Now you build a bar in a doorway a few inches higher than her total height with arms outstretched. You say a little prayer, "Please Lord, let her win just this once!" You are ready to begin.

"Now, honey, I am going to put your hands around this bar and you must hold on for one minute the way all your friends in Philadelphia want you to do. Once you get a grip, I'll let go of you, and it will be just as if you are standing up all by yourself for the first time in your life only your feet won't be touching the floor. Don't worry, honey, because when you can't hold on any longer, I'll catch you, so you don't have to worry. Here we go, honey!"

With your heart in your mouth and a prayer on your lips, you, Mother, open her little hands while your husband supports her weight and you wrap them around the bar.

Now you let go and Mary hangs for exactly one-half second before falling into her father's outstretched arms.

"Oh no, honey," you protest, "that was only one-half a second, and you've got to hang one whole minute. It's so important." To her father, you say, "What are we going to *do?* She *must* hang more than a hundred times that long. How will we ever motivate her to do it?"

Now let's look at that perfectly natural episode from Mary's standpoint. Mary is four years old. Being severely brain-injured, she is very small, as brain-injured children are inclined to be, so she only weighs twenty-six pounds. She has never crawled, crept, hung, stood or walked in her life. She has just tried to hang for the first time in her life and succeeded for only half a second.

"Well," says tiny Mary to herself (being unable to talk), "that's failure six-thousand-four-hundred and ninety-two. I failed again! That's the story of my life."

Mary, being very hurt, may not be able to articulate it quite that clearly, but that is precisely what she'll feel. What else could she *possibly* think under that set of circumstances?

Now suppose we ask ourselves a question. Just how long *should* a paralyzed, speechless, brain-injured four-year-old child with the body of a two-year-old be able to hang from a bar the first time she tries it? How long should *any* little four-year-old girl hang, for that matter?

Well it is obvious that you don't know and neither do I. If we don't know how long she should be able to hang, it is pretty obvious that *she* doesn't. While I don't know that answer in advance for any one little girl, I know without question that for some little girls the first time out one-half second is a very long time to hang.

Now let's suppose that instead of the "Gosh, honey, that just isn't good enough" approach, you had used a different approach.

Suppose at the end of that one-half second when Mary dropped into Dad's arms, you had taken her into your arms and said, "Wow!"

Suppose you had hugged her and kissed her and said, "Who would have *dreamed* that a tiny little girl like *you* could have hung on to that bar for a whole half second?"

Suppose you had told her she was a most extraordinary little girl. Suppose you had told her that she was without question the most remarkable child in the whole city, probably the most magnificent child in the entire state and possibly the best little girl in the whole *world*.

Suppose you had told her with love and with respect.

Suppose also that you *meant* it. Do you know any other little four-year-old girl who can't move and can't talk who ever even *tried* to hang by her hands?

Let's not play games with whether a speechless four-year-old girl understands what it means to be the most remarkable child in all the city. *She'll* understand the real message. When you squeeze her to your breast you'll feel nice and warm and soft and she'll get the message. When she sees the love and the respect on your face for her superb accomplishment, she'll get that message. When she hears the love and respect in your voice, she'll get that message, and she doesn't need to understand a word of English to do so.

We adults make the mistake of listening to each other's words to some degree, and we are thus misled when some other adult chooses to mislead us. But nobody really fools kids because when they are listening for important messages (rather than mere information), they don't really listen to the words. They listen to the music.

Considering the two possible approaches, it's immediately obvious that in *either* case she hung for one-half second. We have no way of knowing whether that's good or bad, really, but we do know this. You may look at what she did from two very different vantage points.

If, in your anxiety to get it right for her own good, you insist on looking at the difference between the way she *is* the first time she tries this new and important treatment and the way you *want* her to be, then you can only bemoan the fact that it is not good enough.

If such is the case, then you must not be surprised when Mary says to herself, "Yep, that's my six-thousand-four-hundred and ninety-second failure, and now the big ones are going to keep at me with this new damned business at which I will now fail as many times a day as they make me do it. It's the story of my life."

And she will.

That's what *I* do.

Now if, on the other hand, what you want is for her to do it again and again and to attack it with enthusiasm and to want to do it again and again, then you might be wise to look at it from the vantage point of where she *was* yesterday and where she *is* today.

Yesterday nobody would have dreamed of asking this immobile and speechless little girl to hang by her hands at all. Today she can support her own weight by hanging from her hands for a full half second. When *you* appreciate the miracle that has happened and show your respect for that accomplishment, then surely Mary will glow with the pleasure of accomplishment and of Mommy's praise and then she will say with or without words:

"Yes, I did do that well, didn't I? Would you like to see me do it again?"

And she will.

That's what *I* do.

And if you *do* want her to do it again so that every day she gets better, until sixty days later when it's time for her revisit to Philadelphia, she can hang for sixty seconds, then I strongly recommend that you appreciate what she *can* do. That's motivation with a capital "M."

It is you, Mother, who *decide* what success or failure is.

If you want to win in making your child well, then look at the difference between where she is and where you want her to be, which is to say the difference between the way she is (hurt) and the way you want her to be (well), but *don't* pound the child's ear about that. That is *your* problem and *mine*. Pointing out how far the child has yet to go makes it sound as if how *far* to go were her fault.

Thus, we have the formula: failure which leads to punishment which leads to lack of motivation which leads to her stubbornly refusing to try. Or as Mary puts it, "That's the story of my life."

If, on the other hand you want to motivate Mary to try and try and try again until she can hang on a bar for a minute or walk or talk or read or write, then it behooves you to look at where she is today versus where she was before you started such an intensive program, which is to say the difference between the way she is and the way she was, and you must be grateful and enthusiastic and respectful and joyous.

Thus we have the formula: success which leads to rewards which leads to motivation which leads to her actually wanting to do it again and looking forward to doing it again. Or, as Mary puts it, "Yes, I did do that well, didn't I? Would you like to see me do it again?"

If you would like to see her do whatever it is again, try rewarding her with your love and praise.

But of course, being a parent, you always knew all of that in your heart and I'm sure that you've almost always practiced it, but I just thought I ought to mention it.

26.

WHO IS BRAIN-INJURED?
WHO IS NOT?

If everyone could simply agree on what is meant by the various terms used to describe brain-injured children, we'd be a long way along the road to solving such problems.

The great American psychiatrist Dr. Menninger, of the Menninger Clinic, once told me that when man encounters a mysterious illness he is inclined to label it, to hang tags on it, because he feels that by doing so he has somehow achieved a degree of mastery over it. Dr. Menninger pointed out that this rarely adds to the clarity but instead adds to the confusion.

Confusion of terminology is certainly a problem in the world of the brain-injured child. That's why this book is entitled, *What to Do About Your Brain-injured Child, or Your Brain-damaged, Mentally Retarded, Mentally Deficient, Cerebral-palsied, Emotionally Disturbed, Spastic, Flaccid, Rigid, Epileptic, Autistic, Athetoid, Hyperactive Child.* Now that, admittedly, is a terrible name for a book, and all you can say is, "What the devil does that mean?"

That is exactly what I'd hope you'd say because that's exactly the question that needs asking. What the devil do all those words mean?

If you are the parent of a brain-injured child, you have surely heard all of these words. It is quite possible that different specialists have given your child most or even all of these names. We see tiny children who have been diagnosed as every one of those things, each in a different institution, and when I look at a tiny two-year-old child I wonder if it is really possible for one little girl to have so many terrible diseases—if diseases they are.

Just what do these terms mean? Are brain-damaged children the same as *mentally retarded* children? Are brain-injured children the same as *mentally deficient* children? Are all such children *emotionally disturbed,* or is that a different problem? What of children with *cerebral palsy?* Is this one kind of condition when the child is bright, and something else when he is mentally retarded? Are all C.P. children *spastic, flaccid, both, or neither?* Always? Sometimes?

Just what do these terms mean? Do they mean what they say? If they don't mean what they say, then what do they mean?

Let's take the term *emotionally disturbed.* Many brain-injured children are diagnosed as being *emotionally disturbed.* What does this term mean? Is it intended to replace *brain injury* as a diagnosis; that is to say, is this child *emotionally disturbed* rather than *brain-injured?* Or is he suffering from two different diseases simultaneously? Just what disease is *emotionally disturbed,* or is it, in fact, a disease at all? What does the term mean? If it means what it *says*—emotionally disturbed—then I can say that I, one of the most fortunate of men, find myself emotionally disturbed twenty or thirty times a day about one thing or another. I have a sneaky suspicion that you do, too. I don't believe that anyone in his right mind could read the front page of any large metropolitan newspaper without being emotionally disturbed over virtually every front-page story. At least he should be emotionally disturbed if *emotionally disturbed* means what it says. On the other hand, if the term *emotionally disturbed* as used to diagnose brain-injured children does not mean what it says, then the overriding question which remains is: What does it mean?

Or let's take what is probably the best known term: *Cerebral Palsy. Cerebral* means *brain* and *palsy* means *paralysis.* To some people *palsy* means *to shake.* Since the brain can neither shake nor be paralyzed, the term *cerebral palsy* clearly does not mean what it says. The question then is—what does it mean?

One great authority on the subject of cerebral palsy has said that cerebral palsy means *a highly specific set of symptoms produced by a highly specific and specifically located type of brain injury.* Fair enough, and that would do for a term and a diagnosis were it not for the fact that another great authority has said that cerebral palsy means a very different thing. He has said that *cerebral palsy is anything that happens to a child from the neck up.* Also fair enough, if it were not for the first authority. Unhappily this disagreement does not end with these two authorities. There are virtually as many different meanings as there are authorities in the field, and there are many authorities.

Nor does refinement of terms necessarily help.

The term cerebral palsy can be broken down into several different sub-categories, one of which is *athetoid cerebral palsy.* In some classifications this term is then broken down further into sub-terms describing ten or twelve types of athetoids. Dr. Fay, who had personally authored or co-authored several classification methods in an early attempt to bring some order out of chaos, used to say rather ruefully that there were actually only two types of athetoids. The two types, Dr. Fay used to say, were "them as had it and them as didn't." That reduced the types of athetoids rather considerably. We come, in the end, to agree with Menninger that "refining the terminology" added to the confusion rather than to the clarification.

The trouble with almost all of the names we have discussed and the many others that exist is every time we use them we are compounding the easy error of mistaking the symptom for the disease.

A good example is the very popular term *mental retardation*. An American today would have to be not only televisionless and radioless, but deaf and blind as well, not to have heard this term over and over again. "*Mental retardation* can strike any home." "Every two minutes a child is born afflicted with *mental retardation*." "Fight *mental retardation*." "Give money for research into the cause of *mental retardation*." "This child is a victim of *mental retardation*."

Doesn't all this leave the impression that there is a disease called *mental retardation*? There is no such disease. Mental retardation is a symptom and, like most other symptoms, is a symptom of many very different diseases. One can have the symptom, mental retardation, because his mother and father have incompatible Rh factors. One can have the symptom, mental retardation, because he got hit by an automobile. One can have the symptom, mental retardation, because he was born with the umbilical cord wrapped tightly around his neck. One can show the symptom, mental retardation, because he had measles, which resulted in encephalitis, and so on through a hundred very different diseases and injuries that can result in the symptom of severe, moderate or mild mental retardation.

To talk about mental retardation as if it were a disease is not only unscientific but, what is more important, seriously delays the finding of rational answers to problems. Because this point is so important, I must risk belaboring it to be sure I have made myself clear. Let's take a clear and fairly precise analogy.

Let's suppose that today someone should announce that he has discovered that seven million Americans have a Fever and that this condition can be as serious as it is mysterious. Suppose that he should announce that this mysterious illness of elevated temperature, or Fever, ranged in effect from a mild inconvenience at one end of the spectrum to actual death at the other and that this very day hundreds of Americans would die afflicted with Fever. Suppose he announced that every eight seconds an American was born who would someday be afflicted with Fever. Suppose finally he announced that he had just found out that there was no American Fever Society and that he was going to raise millions of dollars to organize such a society for the purpose of combating the killer, Fever.

If that should happen, it is to be hoped that someone would say to this man, "Each of the things you have said is true. You are obviously motivated by the highest and most selfless intentions, *but you must not do this*. While each of the things you have said is true, the conclusion you have drawn is untrue. Fever is not a *disease* but is instead a *symptom* of many different and unlike diseases or injuries. If you form such a society you will convince many people, and even some professionals, that there is actually such a disease. This will hide the truth and, in the end, be a disservice to mankind."

This is what has actually happened as a result of the popularization of that very imprecise term, *mental retardation*.

Mental retardation is no more and no less a symptom than is fever; neither symptom is a disease. If one successfully attacks the disease of which fever is a symptom, the fever will disappear spontaneously, as is the case with the symptoms in other diseases. By the same token, if one successfully attacks the brain injury of which mental retardation can be a symptom, the mental retardation will also disappear spontaneously.

How did this term arise and what does it actually mean?

Most people use the term, mental retardation, to describe children who do not learn as quickly or are not able to learn as much as average children. It has come to have an additional meaning which is almost always implied but less often voiced. Mental retardation has the arch implication that it exists in a child because his mother should not have married his father, or that his grandmother should not have married his grandfather. While it is true that the symptom of mental retardation can be present in a child because of the combination of his mother and father, this is true in only a small fraction of the total number of children who have the symptom.

The term mental retardation was coined in an effort at kindliness. So many human problems begin with someone saving someone else from something he hasn't asked to be saved from. Before the term mental retardation was coined as a subterfuge to protect parents from what was considered to be too harsh a truth (harsh it was, truth it was not), we measured intelligence that fell below average (100 being average or normal) and, having done so, we classified sub-normal children into groups according to their scores, and such groups were called morons, idiots or imbeciles.

Since it seemed very harsh to tell a parent that her child was a moron, idiot or imbecile, we invented a euphemism, mental retardation, which term in a literal sense was a splendid choice which labeled the problem quite well. It is what was eventually done with this good but symptomatic term which was the problem. It did not take parents long to come to the conclusion that it was not a compliment to be told that their child was mentally retarded and that what this term really meant was that their child was a moron, idiot or imbecile.

The parents were not fooled, but now we professionals had at least two diseases, idiocy and mental retardation.

It took several years for those who dealt with the parents to come to the conclusion that *mental retardation* meant *idiot* to most parents, and so an even newer term was coined which was an even greater euphemism. This new term to describe children with below-average intelligence was *exceptional*. To call a child with a low I.Q. exceptional was again literally true, but what a splendid euphemism it was. To say that such children were exceptional children rather implied that such children were somehow *better* than other children.

Again the parents were neither flattered nor deceived by such terms. Parents know precisely what their children can and cannot do. Parents very quickly decided that it was not good to be told that their children were exceptional. They decided that what that *really* meant was mentally retarded and what *that* really meant was moron, idiot or imbecile.

Again parents were neither deceived nor mollified, but now we professionals had at least three diseases—idiot children, mentally retarded children and exceptional children.

Mental retardation is not a disease, it is a symptom. *Idiot, emotionally disturbed, flaccid, spastic, quadriplegic, paraplegic, hemiplegic, diplegic,* and a host of other terms by which brain-injured children are called, are all symptoms and none of them are diseases.

We do not believe there are fifty-seven different kinds of children whose problems exist within the brain. We believe that all the children we see can be placed in just three categories. One of these categories we have learned how to help. The other two we have not. Perhaps one day we shall find answers even for the other two.

These three are: (1) the deficient child, (2) the psychotic child, (3) the brain-injured child.

Here is what we mean by each of these groupings.

The Deficient Child: When we at The Institutes in Philadelphia speak of a deficient child, we mean any child who at the instant of conception (not birth) was not intended by the Good Lord or nature to have a good brain. (It must here be pointed out that when we speak of the brain we are not referring to that rather nebulous thing called the mind, but instead to that physical organ that exists inside the skull, that superb collection of living cells that controls all of the bodily functions.)

If one could look at the brain of a deficient child who was never intended to have a good-quality brain, he would see a brain which Fay described as being "composed of little shrunken hairpinlike microgyri instead of the nice, plump, spaghetti-like convolutions which compose a normal brain." This is a brain of bad quality and quantity, and was not destined from the instant of *conception* to be normal.

Of course, it is not always easy to be sure, just from a study of a child's symptoms, whether he has a bad brain or merely a good brain badly hurt. Where we suspect a bad brain, of course, we discuss this frankly with the parents. Such a child is sent to the neurosurgeon for verification. If a question continues to remain, we invariably give the child the benefit of the doubt and give the program a try.

Fortunately, truly deficient children are rare. This much we know from autopsies. There are tens of thousands of children who were diagnosed as deficient, and who lived out their lives in institutions for idiots, but who proved to have been merely brain-injured. I'm afraid there is a fate worse than being a true idiot, and that is to live as an idiot and die as an idiot when you never were an idiot.

In 1967 a story appeared in the American press which told of a child who had been confined to a mental institution for life as an idiot. This particular institutionalized child, however, turned out not to be an idiot. In point of fact, someone discovered that he was, instead, a genius. Although we have not seen this particular child, the odds are heavy that this child was simply brain-injured. Such "little" mistakes are made frequently and will continue to be made until we begin to differentiate between symptoms and diseases in our children with problems. We have seen many, far too many, brain-injured children diagnosed as idiots.

In any event, the truly deficient children have brains of bad quality and quantity, different from the brain-injured children. These are nice children, and they need help, but we have no answers for them. They are, as I have said, rare.

The Psychotic Child: When we speak of a psychotic child, we mean a child whose behavior is markedly different from the normal behavior of other children but whose brain, when seen in the operating room, passes every neurological test or, upon autopsy, appears completely normal even under the microscope.

If there is such a thing as a psychotic brain, as distinct from an injured brain, the difference probably consists in having the brain *improperly* (rather than incompletely) programmed. The tale is told of children adopted from birth by wolves, and nursed and "educated" by wolves, to the point where they behaved like wolves and could never thereafter be re-educated to think of themselves as human beings. Whether the tale is true or false is not the issue. Such children might have had perfectly good brains, yet would certainly have been termed psychotic by human standards.

Since we at The Institutes do not understand "psychotic" children, we have no answers for them. In our considered opinion, however, these children, like the deficient children are, happily, rare.

It is also an unhappy fact that there are thousands of children diagnosed as psychotic who are actually brain-injured and they, too, sometimes live out their lives in mental institutions as if they were insane.

In summary, the truly psychotic children have abnormal behavior but geographically normal brains. They are also rare.

The Brain-injured Child: When we speak of a brain-injured child, we mean any child who, at the instant of conception, *was* intended by nature to have a good brain but who, at some time after that instant of conception, had something happen that hurt that good brain. That something may occur a minute, an hour, a day, a week, a month or nine months after conception. It may occur during birth or a minute, an hour, a day, a week, a month, a year or ten years after birth. It may also happen seventy years after birth, only then he is called a brain-injured adult.

If you could look at this brain in the operating room, you would see a brain of normal quality and you might even be able to see the injury which could consist in highly visible harm confined to a small area, or in harm essentially invisible to the naked eye and spread over a broader area. What is vital here is that it is a *good-quality brain,* hurt. It may be severely hurt or it may be mildly hurt, it may be hurt in a way that limits walking or talking or hearing or seeing or feeling, but it is good-quality brain hurt and not an inferior brain.

These brain-injured children are, like the deficient children and the psychotic children, nice kids and these brain-injured children also need help. We *do* have help and answers for most brain-injured children.

When this book speaks of the brain-injured child, it means that third kind of child alone, and of this kind of child, there are literally millions.

I might paraphrase Abraham Lincoln, and I am sure he would not mind in the least if I said that "God must have loved the brain-injured children because he made so many of them."

27.

HOW MANY BRAIN-INJURED CHILDREN ARE THERE?

The question of how many brain-injured children there may be in this country and abroad may seem of little importance to the parent who already has a brain-injured child. One such child is quite enough for a parent to handle, and knowing how many more there may be in the world may appear to do the parent little good.

However, since many of the Dark Age ideas of the brain-injured child still persist, it may be important for the parent to realize that, in terms of the number of brain-injured children who are actually recognized as being brain-injured, his child is far from alone. If we add the number of brain-injured children, who are not called brain-injured but who are called by any of the several dozen non-specific symptomatic classifications that have been mentioned, then the number becomes very large indeed, and the brain-injured child becomes almost commonplace. If, finally, we should add the number of people who in the technical and scientific sense are brain-injured, that is to say the number of people who have some dead brain cells, we will now find that there are a great many more brain-injured people in the world than there are people who are not brain-injured.

When we at The Institutes meet people who are familiar to some small degree with our work, it is common for them to laugh (a little nervously) and say, "Hey, you know, I'm sure that I must be brain-injured." They are joking, albeit somewhat nervously. The chances are that, in a technical and specific sense, they are right. A top-flight neurophysiologist, McCann, indicates that from thirty-five years of age onward, with each passing day, each of us suffers the death of about one hundred thousand brain cells.

Just how many of us human beings are brain-injured? Due to the almost incredible hodgepodge of terms existing in the jungle of the brain-injured child, it is impossible to know with anything resembling accuracy, but let's take those things we know.

Dr. William Sharpe, the late and prominent New York neurosurgeon, conducted a careful scientific study of five hundred consecutively born newborn children. Within forty-eight hours of their birth, he performed spinal punctures on these children for the purpose of examining their cerebrospinal fluid. (Cerebrospinal fluid is the fluid in which the brain floats. It acts, among other things, to cushion the brain against injury. The cerebrospinal fluid is normally clear and colorless like water.) Dr. Sharpe found that the cerebrospinal fluid taken from *9 per cent* of these presumably normal children contained enough blood to be visible to the naked eye. Dr. Sharpe demonstrated that this was not blood that had been introduced by the puncture of his needle, but instead was blood that was in the cerebrospinal fluid prior to his puncture.

What does this mean? There are many ways to injure the brain which do not put blood in the cerebrospinal fluid, but there is no way to get blood into the cerebrospinal fluid without some break in the internal covering of the central nervous system, in other words an injury.

If Dr. Sharpe's findings in the 1920s could be taken as representative of all newborn children, then we would be forced to the surprising conclusion that a minimum of 9 per cent of all children are demonstrably brain-injured at birth or at least by the time they are two days old.

What has more recent research had to say about such figures? Dr. Sharpe's studies have been repeated many times since, in many different places, and his findings have been confirmed and, what is more, considerably amplified. In later studies, the cerebrospinal fluid was also subjected to microscopic examination. Such studies reveal that from 70–80 per cent of newborn children have some blood cells in the cerebrospinal fluid. Dr. Lewis Jacobs, a New York pediatrician who has in recent years devoted a good deal of time to research in brain-injured children, has told me that, as a young resident a good many years earlier, he had observed such a series of tests done and that, in this particular series, blood was found in the cerebrospinal fluid of 85 per cent of the newborn babies examined. If we can accept such positive findings as being indicative of some very minor injury in 70 per cent of all newborn babies, and of fairly substantial injury (up to and including death itself) in 9 per cent of all children born in the United States, the parent of the brain-injured child can readily see that his strange, brain-injured, different child is not at all strange or different from most other children except in degree.

There is also much research to indicate that the process that ends in senility, namely, the gradual death of individual brain cells, *begins* during childhood and continues at a constantly increasing rate throughout life.

It would be difficult to know how one might define brain injury except as that state in which some portion of the brain's cells are dead. From that point on we are only discussing the number of dead cells. In short, having established the presence of one or more dead brain cells, we are thereafter discussing the *degree* of brain injury rather than whether or not brain injury exists. Under such a definition, it is extremely likely that we can count every human being as brain-injured, at least imperceptibly.

It might seem reasonable to include in a definition of brain-injured only those whose dead brain cells were sufficient in number or location to create recognizable problems, but it is possible that by so doing we shall lose sight of a greater and more important truth.

If you want to see brain-injured people in the truest sense of the word, you need only look around you. If you happen to be alone, you might try looking in a mirror, or, failing that, at my photograph on this book.

28.

WHAT CAUSES BRAIN INJURY?

Brain injury is due to forces from outside the brain itself rather than to any inherent, preconceptual, built-in deficiency. We know of at least a hundred factors that can hurt a good brain subsequent to that instant of conception. There may be a thousand.

In point of fact, it is not terribly important *how* a brain got injured —what counts is how badly and where. Nevertheless, a brain can get hurt in so many ways that it may be worthwhile to review some of them, if only to show that it can happen to anybody.

Among the thousands of brain-injured children who come to The Institutes, we see, for example, the child whose mother and father have an incompatible Rh factor which sets up a blood incompatibility between mother and child. This hurts a good brain.

We see the child whose mother had German measles or some other such contagious disease during the first three months of her pregnancy, or even later in pregnancy. This can hurt a good brain.

We see the child whose mother, during her pregnancy, goes through periods when she doesn't get enough oxygen to supply her needs *and* the baby's.

When I went to school, twenty-five years ago, we were taught that if during pregnancy there was not enough of something to supply the needs of both mother and child, it would be mother rather than child who would suffer. Today we know that it is baby who will get too little. This hurts a good brain.

We see the baby who is born prematurely and who is simply not "done" yet when he is ejected into the world. Until recently babies rarely survived if born prior to the seventh prenatal month, but from the seventh month onward, each additional day makes survival more likely. Of all the factors that may be associated with brain injury, this factor of prematurity comes up most often in our case histories, in fact about three times as often as you would expect purely on the basis of chance. This does not, of course, mean that a premature baby will necessarily be brain-injured, beyond the point that most of us are brain-injured.

We also see more than our share of post-mature babies. Apparently these babies are "too done" as it were, though again (as with most such conditions) the question of what is cause and what is effect is not easy to answer. It is possible that in some of these circumstances it is the brain injury that causes the post-maturity or the prematurity and not the other way round. Nonetheless, we very commonly see these factors associated with hurt children.

We see also the baby whose mother had large amounts of X-ray during pregnancy; even small amounts during the early days can apparently be harmful. Most radiography departments are reluctant to X-ray mothers during pregnancy, particularly during the early days of pregnancy, but this sometimes occurs when Mother is unaware that she is pregnant.

We see also more than our share of children who are born of a precipitous labor, by which we mean a labor lasting less than two hours, or of a protracted labor, by which we mean a labor lasting more than eighteen hours. If either factor is cause rather than effect, then possibly the baby needs a certain time in which to make the violent transition from womb to world—enough time but not too much.

Perhaps because the birth process itself is important, our share of children delivered by Caesarean section is about three times normal. Again there is the possibility that the child may have had to be delivered by Caesarean section *because* he was brain-injured rather than the other way around.

We see, tragically, the baby who is about to be born and whose birth is purposely delayed because the mother has not yet reached the doctor or the doctor has not yet reached the mother. Birth, in these cases we have seen, is generally delayed by having the mother sit up or cross her legs to prevent the baby being born. We have seen so many of these babies that we are completely persuaded that delaying the birth of a baby is a very bad idea. We are persuaded that any nurse, or perhaps even any father, can do a better job of delivering a baby than may result if the birth process is purposely delayed. Recently a friend of ours, Mr. Kurt Gaebel, who is by trade and training one of the world's leading bookbinders (and who not only binds some of our books but who also reads them), was forced to stop en route to the hospital long enough to deliver his own wife of a fine baby in broad daylight in the crowded parking lot of a supermarket. Mother and baby did beautifully although Father remained somewhat shaken for a few days, it being his first delivery. We are persuaded that baby had a better chance of being the fine child it is than would have been the case if the birth had been significantly delayed.

We see also the baby who had obstetrical difficulties due to *placenta previa, placenta abruptio* and other "technical" problems which create difficulties during the birth process. The baby may have been in a position which made his delivery either difficult or even impossible. In such cases, the baby must be manipulated before he can be delivered. In these cases also it is debatable whether the brain injury led to the problem or the problem led to the brain injury.

Long ago, when I went to school, we were given the impression that a high number of brain-injured children were a result of poor obstetrical practices. We have come to believe, however, that this is rare, and that only a very small number of brain-injured children are a result of bad obstetrics. Pre-existing factors in the child frequently make the delivery difficult, thus giving the impression of unnecessarily long delivery.

The brain can also be injured after birth.

We see the infant who at two months of age falls out of a crib or bassinette, causing blood clots on the brain (which are called *subdural hematomas*), and this hurts a good brain.

We see the one-year-old who inhales certain insecticides, which can cause death or very severe brain injury. One of the most severely brain-injured children we have ever seen, who incidentally was one of our relatively small number of *complete* failures, had been a totally normal child until one year of age at which time he had ingested such an insecticide. We have seen other children, brain-injured as a result of poisoning, who have done very well.

We see the four-year-old who falls in a swimming pool and dies of drowning, but who is then revived and who, during the short period of death, was not getting oxygen to his brain and who is brain-injured as a result.

We see the six-year-old who suffers measles or some other infectious disease or who has encephalitis with a very high temperature and who, as a result, is brain-injured.

We see the nine-year-old who, during surgery for tonsilitis or some other problem, sustains a cardiac arrest and dies on the operating table and is revived by open chest surgery and heart massage or some other technique but who during the time when his heart was not beating, like the child who drowned, did not get enough oxygen to the brain and who, as a result, had his good brain injured.

We see the twenty-year-old girl, who in the hours following the birth of her own baby, has a blood vessel rupture in her own brain giving mother, rather than baby, a stroke. If you have an idea that only old people have strokes, we can tell you that the youngest stroke case we ever saw at The Institutes was two months old and that the oldest stroke case we ever saw was 97 years old.

I should not like to leave the impression that young mothers often have strokes following birth. This is not common, but neither is it rare, and it is another way to hurt a good brain—in this case, Mother's.

We see the twenty-year-old who, on the battlefield, gets a bullet through his brain—but I have already told you of my three friends who each got a bullet through the brain. I have also told you how well they did with millions of brain cells not only dead but gone—blown all over the battlefields of Germany and Korea and Belgium. Still it is not a good idea to get a bullet through the brain, and that's another way to hurt a good brain.

We see the thirty-year-old who goes through the windshield in an automobile accident, and that's another way to hurt a good brain.

We see the forty-year-old who has a brain tumor, and that's another way to hurt a good brain.

We see the fifty-year-old who is assaulted with a blackjack in a robbery, and that's another way to hurt a good brain.

We see the sixty-year-old who gets Parkinson's disease, and that also hurts the brain.

We see the ninety-year-old who has literally billions, not merely millions, of cells dead for no better reason than the fact that he's getting pretty old.

All the people described above, and many more, are truly brain-injured people, which is no more than to say that they have a good-quality brain which has a great many dead cells.

But so, on the other hand, do I. It is just that at this moment in history I do not have as many.

29.

THE PAST, PRESENT AND FUTURE
OF THE BRAIN-INJURED CHILD

When the final chapter in the long history of brain-injured children is someday written, there will have been four eras in the story.

THE FIRST ERA—DESPAIR

The first era is happily dead and forever gone. It extended from the earliest beginning of man almost to the beginning of the twentieth century. It was the era of despair. It was marked by cruelty, insanity, and what is perhaps worst of all, secrecy.

The first era had no heroes.

Certainly we do not have to go far back in man's history to find a time when brain-injured children were simply put to death, and we can still see this happening today among the primitive Xingu Indians in the heart of Brazil's Mato Grosso. Terrible and primitive as such a solution may be, it might be considered to be a kindness compared with some of the other solutions that occurred during this, the longest and the most awful era in the story of the brain-injured child. There have been periods—extending up to the eve of the twentieth century—when such hurt children have been tortured for the amusement of unhurt adults. In other periods they have been imprisoned under the most cruel circumstances. They have been starved and they have been beaten.

Under the very best of circumstances, they have been considered a vengeance visited on parents by the Lord as retribution for the sins —either real or fancied—of the parents.

As such, the brain-injured child was a source of shame to his parents and was hidden away in an institution, a back room or an attic so that no one might see their shame, yet throughout the first and most terrible of the four eras of the brain-injured child this was the most benign and kindly of attitudes. Nor did such an attitude disappear entirely with the coming of the second era.

I can remember as a child during the late nineteen-twenties that there was, in the neighborhood where I lived, a severely brain-injured child of about ten. I know now that this girl had the type of brain injury that is today called athetoid cerebral palsy and that she was very severely involved indeed. I know this today, but I did not, of course, know it then. This child was the daughter of the local pharmacist and this man had the extraordinary courage to put her outside in a carriage daily so that she might have some sunshine and fresh air, as she lay totally paralyzed and twisted in her oversized baby carriage. He had the courage to do so, but he paid the price for his courage.

I remember that the children accepted her quite naturally as she lay in her carriage, as much a part of her surroundings as the drugstore itself. I am sure the children would have paid her no attention at all and would have come to the conclusion that such a child was a natural part of every drugstore in the land, in much the same way that a red-and-white barber pole stood outside every barber shop, had it not been for the adults in the neighborhood.

It is frequently said that children are cruel, like animals, and savage, like, well, like savages, toward other children and especially toward hurt children. If there is any truth at all in this idea, it is only true after adults have taught them to be cruel. Children are not born full of fears, prejudices and supersititions. They are taught those things, and we adults are the teachers. Children are born with total acceptance of the way things are. Skies are blue, some kids have red hair, some kids have green eyes, some kids can run fast and some kids can't move. They learn to question why these things are so as quickly as they learn to talk, but they accept as total truth whatever answers adults give them. They also learn without asking questions, by simply listening to what adults say to each other, and what most of the adults said about our neighborhood brain-injured child was cruel, untrue and ignorant in its content and worse in its implications. The child, it was said, was a monster and anyone would think that "they" would have enough decency not to let the sight of her offend the eyes of decent people. The least they could do was to "put her (or it) away." It was implied that such monsters were no accident, and normal, healthy families did not produce such children. What kind of diseased or twisted mind or heritage would parents have to have to produce such an offense to the community? Such a disease would have to be a dirty disease which must have its roots in sex and, moreover, run in the family.

One occasionally still hears such talk today, but today, thanks to the heroes of the second era, such filthy superstition is the exception rather than the rule. When I was a boy in the nineteen-twenties it was the rule rather than the exception, and I was raised in a "nice middle-class neighborhood." My neighborhood was not exceptional and people are little different today than they were then. What happened in my neighborhood was simply a reflection of the pathetic ignorance of the time in relation to brain-injured children.

THE SECOND ERA—DISCOVERY

The second era in the story of the brain-injured child was the era of discovery. It was a happier era, and if it did little to solve the disabilities of the brain-injured child, and if it made a great many mistakes as to treatment, it did many things of inestimable value, among which were the vital accomplishments of bringing the brain-injured child into the blessed light of day, making it respectable to discuss his problems. The second era is still very much alive today.

The second era had a handful of very great heroes as well as thousands of less-heroic and less-brilliant followers. While many of these courageous leaders are now gone and have taken their proper place in the history of those who have contributed to man's progress, others of them remain alive today to receive the homage due them.

These great men were innovators. They had come to make changes in the way things were, and man has never taken kindly to great changes or to the innovators who insist on such changes. Perhaps it is well that this is so. New ideas, however logical or however true, must ever be exposed to the harsh light of scientific question in the continuous quest for truth so that what is dishonest, untrue, specious or spurious may be weeded out. In the end, the truth will defend itself.

However, the light of scientific question is hard on what is false and what is true alike. This harsh light falls not only on the innovation but also, and more particularly, on the innovator, be he charlatan or genius. Not all innovators have had the courage to withstand the harsh but necessary treatment which all innovators receive, and many who have espoused important truths have wilted and run from such investigations when their courage did not match the value of the truths they offered. When such has been the case, such truths have been re-buried to await rediscovery by people whose brilliance in unearthing truth was matched by the strength and courage needed to defend it.

These heroes of the second era had courage to match their beliefs. Their way was not easy. The battle that these men fought was not against an organized and ruthless foe who defended a different view. They had no such easy task. Such an enemy is visible and, however formidable he may be, he can be seen, identified and therefore attacked. The giants who introduced the second era had a much more subtle, difficult and elusive enemy. This enemy was supersitition, folklore and indifference. The goal of the leaders of the second era was clear and simple. They wanted to make the world aware that brain-injured children are just that, children who are brain-injured. Not monsters, not objects of shame or ridicule, but children pure and simple. Children who are like many other children, hurt, but hurt in the brain rather than with broken arms or appendicitis. Today this may seem pathetically clear and simple. Today it may seem obvious, but it wasn't then. Remember my druggist.

The enemies—superstition, folklore and indifference—were everywhere but they were also nowhere. How does one fight an enemy he can neither identify nor see? There are few more infuriating, frustrating and difficult battles to be fought than those whose enemy is almost total apathy. One must first find his enemy; he must then make his enemy aware that he is the enemy (for who admits superstition, indifference or belief in folklore, even to himself?); and then he must make the enemy defend himself. Only then can he begin an honest fight. All these were the problems faced by the heroes of the second era. They fought these problems and they fought them well and in the end, although it took nearly half a century, they won. Fifty years may seem a very long time to win such a clear and simple point—unless you consider the hundreds of thousands of years of ignorance that preceded it.

Although there were a very few others prior to the turn of the century, perhaps we can begin the second era, the Era of Discovery, with a physician named William John Little, 1810–94. Dr. Little was a British surgeon who described the *congenital spastic diplegic,* paralyzed in both legs.

While Dr. Little's work with the brain-injured child served to make physicians aware that such children should at least be diagnosed, and provided physicians with a name by which to call such children (they were now called Little's Disease), his work did little or nothing to bring such children to the attention of the general public.

By the nineteen-thirties and the early nineteen-forties the names of the more successful heroes of the second era, the ones who made it stick, began to be heard and known to many physicians and to many parents. Those names were Winthrop Phelps, Temple Fay, Meyer Pearlstein and a dozen others in the United States, England and elsewhere.

These men had fought a noble and courageous battle against difficult odds to make the public aware that the brain-injured child was hurt and needed and deserved help. They fought and they won.

In their wake came public awareness, physician interest, the formation of professional groups to study the problem of brain-injured children, as well as lay groups which collected funds for treatment and research and for public education. All these were huge steps in the right direction. All of them made both scientists and lay people aware that this problem existed and that something should and must be done about it.

As a result of these societies and of increased public awareness, treatment centers followed in their wake. By the time of World War II, a very few treatment centers were in existence, such as Dr. Phelps' Institute for Brain-Injured Children in Maryland and Dr. Fay's Neurophysical Rehabilitation Center in Philadelphia. By the year 1950, there were a few more inpatient institutes for treatment of brain-injured children in this nation, and outpatient treatment centers had sprung up in almost every state. By 1960 there were hundreds.

All this was a very necessary step in the right direction and was made possible by the few courageous pioneers who had arisen to meet this problem.

The names of Phelps and Fay are justifiably famous. Without such men there would not be the rest of us or the work this book describes. They are our personal heroes.

Those of the original pioneers who are still alive, are honored teachers, professors and practitioners. Having survived their own days as innovators and pioneers they have remained to reap the rewards of honor and respect they have so justly earned. Students flock to their doors from all over the world to learn and pay homage. This is exactly as it should be. These men have earned their place in history, a history which those of us who have followed will write and are even now writing.

As is natural and proper, these men are also today the arbiters of *what* is right and wrong and *who* is right and wrong in their world of the brain-injured child. The circle has come around. The former pioneers, radicals and innovators have now grown respectable and deeply respected since the truths that they espoused have been made obvious and, therefore, respectable.

However, during the second era, when so many, many things had to be accomplished and so many things remained undone, it was inevitable that some of the answers which came into being should be partial answers, incomplete answers or even sometimes no answers at all. This was true of the second era in terms of treatment itself. The second era did not propose that the goal of treatment was or should be to make the brain-injured child *well*. Such a goal was considered to be not only highly improbable but more than that, impossible. To talk of making a brain-injured child well was considered to be not only dangerous and highly irresponsible but, what was worse, downright silly. There were few if any of the second era who would be willing to accept such talk even as a future and some-day goal. To make a brain-injured child well seemed clearly, to almost everyone, to be a contradiction in terms. However, such talk was seldom a problem in the heyday of the second era of the brain-injured child since, if there were none of the leaders who would listen to such wild talk, there were very few who would dare to have such thoughts and virtually none who dared to voice such radical ideas.

Man frequently does not succeed in attaining the objectives he sets for himself—and he very rarely attains *higher* objectives than those he seeks. Since making brain-injured children well was not even a goal of the second era, it was not accomplished, and brain-injured children did not get well.

If wellness was not the goal of treatment during the second era, it is reasonable to ask what the goals were.

The goals were actually three in number. The first was to prevent the child's symptoms from becoming worse and, where possible, to lessen such symptoms as spasticity, tightening of heel cords or the deformity of joints. The treatment that had been pioneered by the leaders of the second era frequently succeeded in preventing the worsening of these symptoms, and it sometimes, although not too often, succeeded in the reduction of such symptoms.

The second goal of treatment was to fit the child into his world better by altering his environment so that he could live more easily or more successfully as a cripple. As an example, if a child could not walk due to his brain injury, he might be able to achieve some degree of independence in a wheel chair if he could manipulate such a wheel chair with his hands and if his home could be altered to replace steps with ramps. While the example I have used is simple, such methods were frequently ingenious and highly engineered.

The third goal of treatment was to teach the brain-injured child anything he seemed capable of learning within the limitations imposed by his brain injury. Thus, the brain-injured child who could not function might be taught to feed himself with spoons twisted into unusual shapes to counteract his deformities, or with a spoon strapped onto his hand. If the child was able to learn to count, to recite poetry, to read or to write, he was provided with teaching so that he might improve, to the highest point possible, whatever skills he had.

It is quite clear that the second era offered the brain-injured child and his parents circumstances far superior to those of the first era. It was so obviously better for the brain-injured child to have his symptoms lessened rather than increased. It was better for him to be able to move around in a wheel chair than not to be able to move around at all. It was better for a child to be able to feed himself with a special spoon strapped on his hand than not to be able to feed himself at all. There is no question that the second era offered the brain-injured child a life far superior to the tortures of the first era. The new life fell far, far short of normality, however, and almost as far short of happiness or usefulness. It in no way solved the parents' problem of what, in the end, was going to happen to their child.

The whole treatment concept of the second era was based on the assumption that to attack his symptoms was the best thing to do since there would be no way of attacking the problem where it actually existed, in the brain itself. That basic assumption remained unchallenged through many years of era two, and brain-injured children did not get well.

It was astonishing that the basic assumption that nothing could be done about the brain itself should remain unchallenged for almost half a century of modern times and modern medicine. It was inevitable that it would one day be challenged, and I believe it was our group who first seriously challenged this notion.

Interestingly enough, it was Temple Fay himself, one of the great leaders of the second era, who was becoming daily more disenchanted with the lack of positive results, who laid the groundwork for the ultimate destruction of the second era and planted the seeds for the establishment of the third era. Fay, who had been a cofounder of the

Academy of Cerebral Palsy, and who, with Phelps, had been largely responsible for the successes of the second era, had two serious complaints about what was happening. First, he complained that what was happening was helpful but, to a large degree, unmedical. He pointed out repeatedly that the traditional role of medicine was to seek out and attack the damaged or diseased part itself and to seek to repair it rather than to teach people how best to live with a disability. He strongly questioned whether teaching people how to live with a disability was the role of modern medicine or at the least whether this should remain the primary objective.

Fay complained, secondly, that although brain-injured children were clearly neurological problems, the treatment they were receiving was almost entirely orthopedic. He pointed out that we could not hope to solve a neurological problem by orthopedic treatment. Fay also conceded that this was due in large part to the fact that in the early nineteen-forties very few neurologists or neurosurgeons demonstrated much real interest in the problems of brain-injured children. Since Fay himself was both a neurologist and a neurosurgeon who had earned an international reputation in those fields, he was eminently qualified to voice such an opinion.

Fay's genius, indeed Fay's mere presence on our team, could not help but draw our attention away from the brain-injured child's symptoms which existed everywhere in the child's body from his toes to his eye, and to direct our attention to the brain itself where the child's real problem actually existed. It is simultaneously ironic and highly proper that Dr. Fay, a pioneer of the second era, should also have been the inspiration, if not the prime mover, for its eventual destruction.

It is difficult to know when the third era began. Certainly the seeds were planted by 1941, as we, Fay's students, began to ponder the implications of his emphasis on the relation of brain injury and bodily dysfunction.

Certainly his presence on the team and the role of leadership he played from 1945 until 1957 were vital. Fay's vast knowledge of how the brain functioned, as well as his many theories as to how we might approach treatment were invaluable in bringing about the third era, although at the time we were unable to achieve much in the way of practical results.

I do not know just when the third era began. Perhaps it began in our minds in 1941, without our awareness that it existed. Its theories were surely evolving in our awareness by 1950. By 1955 we were quite aware of the necessity for the third era. By 1960 we had announced the third era to those colleagues who chose to listen, and by 1965, although the second era was still very much alive, the third era was definitely in being and obviously here to stay.

THE THIRD ERA—RATIONAL TREATMENT

While the second era attacked the symptoms of the brain-injured child and had as its goal the prevention of deformity, the lessening of symptoms and the adroit fitting of the child into his environment, the third era is the era of rational and successful *treatment* of the brain-injured child. The third era attacks the brain itself where the problem lies and the objective of such treatment is not to make the child a happy or successful cripple but instead to make him a noncripple, in both physical and intellectual terms.

I wish that I could now report that we are presently able to do this successfully with all children who seek treatment. This, of course, is not the case, but it *is* the case that we are making *some* brain-injured children completely well and even some severely brain-injured ones completely well. The majority of brain-injured children we are seeing today are markedly and measurably improved.

It is hardly astonishing that we should sometimes fail to make brain-injured children well in a world which by and large still believes that such an objective is an impossibility. It should be surprising that we sometimes succeed.

By the beginning of the third era, the innovators, radicals and pioneers of the second era had become the respected leaders of the world of brain-injured children as well as its guardians and arbiters, and a new group of radicals, innovators and pioneers had come forth to demand to be heard and to add their new knowledge, ideas and energy to the war on brain injury.

Who were these new dissidents? Fay was certainly one of them as was the team of younger men Fay had inspired and led.

However, if I have given, up to now, the impression that we were the only ones who were dissatisfied with the results being obtained, I must hasten to correct this view, for such is not the case. While those who were looking for better methods of treatment did not necessarily agree with each other, they did have one thing in common. They were all looking away from limbs and orthopedics and toward the nervous system and neurology. Most of these innovators had stopped talking of "musculoskeletal disorders" and now spoke of "neuromuscular disorders." Such a view, if it did not entirely abandon the symptoms and the muscles, had at least made a distinct move toward the human central nervous system and thus the cause.

While Deaver and Phelps still clung to muscles and bracing as the answer, others such as Knott, Kabat, Rood, Ayers and Semans were advocating either various neuromuscular techniques or the use of neurological reflexes, which Fay had urged as early as the late nineteen-thirties and which we had used in 1941 and advocated in the immediate post-war years.

Others had gone even farther from the musculoskeletal symptoms and were actually looking to the brain itself for answers. These people included the Bobaths, Brunnstrom, Wind and others, both in this country and abroad.

It is quite difficult to know how to deal fairly with the third era and its cast of characters at this particular point in history since this is a highly transitional time.

While most of the world continues to *treat* the brain-injured child by the symptom attack of the second era, a majority of the world is dissatisfied with the old techniques and at least half of the world is presently seeking to learn about the new methods so that they can begin to utilize them. Greater numbers are daily looking in the direction of the new methods. However, at this time there remain the advocates of the old methods (some are violent in their advocacy) and there are the advocates of the new methods (some also violent in their advocacy). This presents a real problem in reporting the coming of the third era, with due recognition to those responsible for its coming.

If I should assume that we at The Institutes for the Achievement of Human Potential are solely responsible for the coming of the third era, I shall surely be attacked by many advocates of the third era for taking undue credit.

If, on the other hand, I give due credit to the others who have purposely or even unconsciously played an important role in bringing about the third era, I shall unquestionably be attacked by some advocates of the second era for trying to spread the blame for something which they consider to be radical, controversial and perhaps, in their opinions, even full of dangerous new ideas. So, unquestionably, in some quarters I shall be damned if I do and damned if I don't. These are invariably the problems of all people who have something new to say that runs contrary to the ideas the present day cherishes. In addition to the people who line up clearly on either side of an issue, there are always a great number who stand in the middle, who cannot make up their minds and who want the comfort of both while denying the responsibility for either. Their argument generally runs that the new ideas are new, dangerous, silly and unproven and, besides all that, these ideas are not new and they have always done them that way anyhow. Such fence straddlers always remind me of the Army recruit who writes home that Army food isn't fit for pigs, in addition to which you get such small servings.

I shall solve my dilemma by reporting the third era and its people exactly as it and they appear to me, and in so doing assume the role of a reporter who, while much involved in his subject, is doing his level best to report the happenings as they appear to him.

To do so, I herewith absolve completely from blame for our ideas anyone who wishes to disassociate himself from such ideas while simultaneously acknowledging the complete contributions of anyone who has contributed, whether I am aware or unaware of his contribution, as well as welcoming to his place in the third era all those who choose to be associated with it whether they have contributed much, little or nothing except their own accord to its existence. I do all of the above while remaining completely responsible for our own contributions, ideas and work.

While my group does not claim complete credit (or blame) for the third era, it is safe to say that we have been an important part of it from its earliest beginnings.

Where does the third era now stand? Most children in the world are still being treated by the methods of the second era, although today many thousands of other children in dozens of nations on all continents are being treated by the methods developed by The Institutes, while thousands more are being treated by the neurological methods espoused by the Bobaths, by Brunnstrom, Rood, Knott and others who are, in our opinion, an important part of the third era.

Many of the leaders of the second era have become convinced that the new methods have something of value to offer the brain-injured child and are using the new methods in part or in full. Others hold tightly to the old method, but the tide is swinging, and swinging rapidly.

Students and post-graduate practitioners from all of the fields concerned in the treatment of the brain-injured child still flock to the respected leaders of the second era, as they properly should and as we ourselves had done, although there is some feeling that such journeys

today are compounded less out of the need to learn than out of the
desire to pay homage to some of medicine's greats.

Of the students still going in large numbers to learn from and pay
homage to the leaders of the second era, many are going as well to
those who advocate the new methods of the third era.

Time was when mention of The Institutes raised only eyebrows in
some circles. Today, such mention, as like as not, draws enthusiastic
comment from individuals who have actually been patterners. Thousands of physicians now refer children for treatment. Over a hundred
have put their own brain-injured children on the program. Scientific
seminars now rarely discuss the old techniques but are almost entirely
devoted to the methods and the proponents of the new third era.

In sum, the third era and its people are becoming respectable. We
are becoming a little more conservative. It is to be hoped that we
do not too quickly become too conservative because complete con-
servativeness almost always brings with it a closing of the mind to
new ideas.

It now seems certain that the ideas of the third era will replace
the second entirely, and when they do, its advocates will assume
their new positions of complete respectability, and eventually reverence, and will themselves become the arbiters of what is right and
what is wrong and, as such, the sole custodians of the truth as they
see the truth. It is probable that we of The Institutes will be numbered
among these people. If that day comes, I am sure that we, like the
others before us, will completely enjoy such veneration and prominence, and the third era will have fulfilled its promise. If that day
comes when we are considered right instead of always wrong, it is
likely that we will then be held to be *always* right, even when we're
wrong.

Then one day, the fourth, final and best era of the brain-injured
child will begin.

THE FOURTH ERA—PREVENTION

It will probably begin with a new and unheard of group of angry
young people in Upper Tomahawk, Kansas, or San José, Brazil, who
will probably say, with fine disregard for proper reverence, "Those
old jugheads in Philadelphia (and elsewhere) have not had a new
idea about brain-injured children in twenty years." They will probably go on to say, "Those old gents were fine in their day, but they are
wrong in their basic assumption that the best thing to do about brain-

injured children is to make them well; it was all right twenty years ago but it's no good today." Then they are surely going to say, "The real answer to brain-injured children is not to cure them but to prevent them."

Those young people, of course, will be absolutely right. Those young people will not only be right in what they say (many people, including us, are already saying it), but what is much more important, they'll know how to do it. Probably at first they will not know how to prevent all brain-injured children but only some of them, but as they continue, the numbers they will be able to prevent will continue to grow.

Those young people will probably say of us, "We love and respect those old gentlemen in Philadelphia and we are for giving them parades, medals, professorships, awards and the place they have earned in history." They will also add ominously, "But we are not in favor of sacrificing a single child to them." In this, too, they will be absolutely right.

We sometimes find a few minutes (generally at two or three A.M.) to think about that future day and discuss it. We know it will come and pray for its coming, for it will be a glorious day for the world. We like to think that when that day does come we will say, "Listen to these young men and women because they are unquestionably right." We like to believe that when that day comes we will not only agree with them but will rally whatever influence or prestige we may then have behind them. We like to believe that by joining them, we, like Fay, will have the golden opportunity to be part of two eras in the history of the brain-injured child. If we do, they will welcome us with open arms and learn from us, as we welcomed and learned from the truly great Dr. Temple Fay.

We like to believe all that, but we are also students of history and realists to boot. The odds are against us doing so, and we know it. Unhappily, history and the odds indicate that when those young people arrive on the scene we will say, "It is young people like these, full of wild impossible ideas and given to overstatement, who cause all the trouble in the world," and thus proceed to condemn them for threatening all the ideas we fought so long and so hard to establish.

We vow we shall *not* do this, but history testifies that we will. We often talk about putting a letter in the safe addressed to ourselves to be reopened and reread on the first of every new year. This letter will say, "Are there any young people around who are giving us a particularly

bad time who just might be right?" We often talk about writing such a
letter, but it seems more than a little interesting that we have not yet
done so. I wonder if that means anything?

In the off chance that we never do get around to writing that letter,
then let this book serve as my accolade to and full acceptance of that
future group of young men and young women.

1970 to 1980
THE DECADE OF THE WELL KIDS

Susan Aisen
Ann Ball
Barbara Barstow
Maxwell Britt
Frank Caputo
Janet Caputo
Leia Coelho
Rose Craddock
Adelle Davis
Helen Derr
Robert Derr
Douglas Doman
Joseph Gay
Bruce Hagy
Stanley Holt
Masaru Ibuka
Vanessa Ingram
Fumikatsu Inoue
Professor Isao Ishii
James Kaliss
Mary Kett

Rosalind Klein
Phyllis Kimmel
Grace Luft
Claire Mapow
Kaname Matsuzawa
James McGeehan
Daniel Melcher
Margaret Melcher
Sam Metzger
Miki Nakayachi
Dawn Price
Judy Reif
Gloria Rittenhouse
Marilyn Rogers
Susumu Samoto
Jerry Schwartz
Dorothy Spady
Professor Shinichi Suzuki
Lidwina van Dyk
Teruki Uemura

30.

THE END OF THE BEGINNING

I date the end of the beginning from that day in May of 1971, when a letter came from Dr. Samarão Brandão, Presidente, da Associadão Brasileiro de Paralisia Cerebral.

Dr. Brandão most cordially invited me to be the principal speaker and the guest of honor of the Fourth Brazilian Congress of Cerebral Palsy of which he was the *presidente* and Dr. Raymundo Araujo Leitão was the *secretario*. Dr. Brandão is a leading orthopedic surgeon of Brazil as well as a physiatrist, while Dr. Leitão is professor of neurological physiatry at the Neurological Institute of the University of Brazil. He is also the author of the leading Brazilian textbook on cerebral palsy.

The Association was the most distinguished medical body in Brazil and was composed primarily of physiatrists, pediatricians, neurologists, orthopedic surgeons and neurosurgeons. The paramedical services were also represented.

The invitation meant a great many things. Many of the people within the Congress represented other groups who had opposed Dr. Veras' doing our work in Brazil. The fact that I was to be the principal speaker could have indicated only that Brazilian professionals wanted to know first hand what I had to say about the work we had carried on for more than thirty years. However, the fact that I was the guest of honor meant far, far more. If the invitation did not mean that the philosophy, concepts, methods and techniques of The Institutes were the *only* ones accepted by Brazilian medical and professional people, it did at least mean that our work was fully recognized in Brazil and was one of the principal methods with full acceptance in that nation.

I wished desperately that Mae Blackburn could have been around to enjoy this break-through in professional acceptance of our methods —she and Jay Cooke and General White and Dr. Sigmund LeWinn and Mr. Henshaw and General Kemp and A. Vinton Clarke and

Eleanor Borden and Betty Marsh and all the others who had shared
the dream and fought the fight and stood fast in the face of failure,
adversity and criticism and who had never, up to the moment of their
deaths, wavered in their determination to find better worlds for
brain-injured kids, and I thought of terms that suited:

> *"We few, we happy few, we band of brothers"*

I thought of others:

> *"Theirs was a royal brotherhood of death"*

And more:

> *"Here was a man, take him all in all,*
> *We shall not see his like again."*

But mostly I thought of Temple Fay and how he would have rel-
ished this day of recognition in Rio de Janeiro.

The Congress itself, which took place the second week of Novem-
ber 1971 at the Copacabana Hotel in Rio de Janeiro, strongly
increased my feeling that our philosophy was widely accepted and
widely used throughout Brazil.

During the sixties the techniques pioneered by The Institutes
were used to some extent, whether well or badly, in a majority of
treatment facilities in the United States, but often on a bootlegged basis. That is to say, our techniques were being used to one degree or
another virtually everywhere in the United States, though many a
user was afraid to acknowledge this. (The department head used
them but did not admit so to the chief of physical medicine, and so
on.)

What a switch Brazil turned out to be! More than five hundred
people registered to take the course in The Institutes' work. Attending were doctors from Brazil, Ecuador, Venezuela, Argentina, Spain,
Peru, the United States and other countries.

Quite literally, hundreds of people sought me out to tell me privately as well as publicly that in their institutions they used *only* the
techniques of The Institutes. I was immensely thrilled and flattered,
but as more and more people told me this I began to be at first slightly
uneasy and then completely suspicious. Was it possible that everyone
in all of Latin America used only our techniques? It seemed unlikely.
So I began to inquire more deeply.

It was clear that a great many people and institutions had come
around to our way of thinking under the influence of those who had
studied with us, notably Drs. Raymundo Veras, José Carlos Veras,
Ivan Porto, Raymundo Arauja Leitão, Raymundo Fontes-Lima and
others in Brazil. It was also abundantly clear that Dr. Eduardo

Sequeiros in Argentina and Dr. Antonio Silva in Peru, after being trained by Dr. Raymundo Veras in Brazil, had taught many others in their own nations and other nations. Our philosophy was clearly widely known and widely practiced in Latin America, but it was equally clear that there were many others who said that they used our methods but who had insufficient knowledge to do so.

How political times do change and how the sands of professional opinion do shift with favorable winds! Whereas before many people had used our techniques while swearing that they did not, now there were some who swore that they did while in truth they did not.

The Institutes had long enjoyed the love and respect and the trust of parents, and this The Institutes had always sought to have and to deserve.

Now The Institutes had the respect and admiration of the professional people of a continent and this it had many years earlier stopped seeking since the earlier price of professional acceptance had been to abandon our work.

We were in.

An additional report made at this Congress strengthened our position even further. I had heard vaguely about it a couple of years earlier.

Toward the end of 1969 the *presidente* (Señora Martinez) of an Argentinian foundation (Da Fundacao Obrigado) had approached Dr. Eduardo Sequeiros, the medical director of The Institutes for the Achievement of Human Potential in Buenos Aires, with a proposal. There was in the city of Córdoba in Argentina a large rehabilitation institute that used classical methods in treating a large number of children. The staff of this institute were convinced that they were achieving no results with their most severe cases, and questionable results with less-severe cases. They had heard about The Institutes' program and wanted to do a study using The Institutes' methods to see if better results might be obtained. This institute was also supported by APANE (Parents Association of Exceptional Children).

Dr. Sequeiros had consulted Dr. Veras in Brazil and they agreed to such a study, imposing two conditions.

1. All staff members of the Córdoba Institute who would work with the children to be tested would be thoroughly trained by Dr. Sequeiros in Buenos Aires and would treat the children in the test group under the direct supervision of Dr. Eduardo Castellani, the medical director of the Córdoba Institute. Dr. Castellani himself would be trained personally by Dr. Sequeiros.

Therefore, the children under treatment by The Institutes' method would be treated *only* by the physicians, psychologists, physical therapists, speech therapists, social workers, etc., of the Cordoba unit with none of the personnel of The Institutes for the Achievement of Human Potential involved.

2. The treatment group would consist only of children who had been on classical methods of treatment for a substantial period of time *and who had failed to show any improvement whatsoever.*

Dr. Castellani decided to make his report to the Congress in the form of a motion picture showing what had occurred to the children after one year of treatment. There was, however, a large problem. Everyone at the institution in Córdoba who had been involved in the experiment wanted to come to Rio with him. The modest budget could not cover thirty-five international plane fares.

A happy solution was achieved. Señora Martinez, the foundation *presidente,* is a wealthy woman, loved and admired by all for her incredible energy and total devotion to brain-injured children. She rented a bus, and thirty-five staff members, Señora Martinez herself and Dr. Castellani drove three days and three nights to attend the Congress.

Their film report was fascinating. Their objective in the study had been simple: to see if any child in a group of fifty who had failed to show *any* improvement on a protracted program of traditional treatment would show any improvement on the program of The Institutes for the Achievement of Human Potential.

They considered the results to be little short of astonishing. *Every* child on the program had shown some improvement. Many had shown extremely important improvement, and some had shown astonishing improvement.

I had used my first three teaching days to cover:
  1. Measurement of the brain-injured child.
  2. Philosophy of treatment of the brain-injured child.
  3. Treatment techniques.

On the last day I had determined to present precisely what had happened to a group of children on the program of The Institutes in Philadelphia.

I had heard Dr. Leitão, professor of physical medicine of the Neurological Institute of the University of Brazil, beginning his final introduction of me.

". . . The people of The Institutes for the Achievement of Human Potential who have endured the criticism and sometimes outright hostility of those of us who are their colleagues, claim to have developed a system of treatment by neurological organization. But we are aware that this is not true. The truth is that these people have pioneered the entire field of neurological rehabilitation and are alone responsible for having told us first in all the world that brain injury is in the brain and that if we are to treat brain-injured people with any hope of success it is the brain itself that we shall have to treat. They have shown us over and over again that this is possible and how it is possible."

It was fortunate that I knew what I was going to say initially, because my eyes were too misted to follow my notes. The essentials of the report I presented to that Congress constitutes the remainder of this chapter. I began:

"MEO CAROS AMIGOS E COLEGOES: We have all of us come through a most trying and difficult number of years. For myself it is more than thirty years. It was, I suppose, inevitable that those years should be marked not only by search, by discovery and by reward, but also by quarrels, by recriminations, by attacks and by defenses since man has always been fearful of change. Yet it must be equally obvious to all of us that the mighty problems which face the children of the world and consequently all of us, do not allow even a moment for family quarrels. The past has clearly failed the brain-injured child and his parents. Let us today bury the past with its recriminations forever. Surely we are no longer helpless.

"During this week you have heard from the two Maggies. Margaret Rood is my friend, and she speaks to you of neurology. It must be clear to you that she has something of value for the children of the world. For the children's sake let us *use* it and bury a non-productive past.

"During this week you have also heard from Margaret Knott. She is my friend, and she speaks to you of neurology. It must be clear to you that she has something of value for the children of the world. For the parents' sake let us *use* it and bury a past in which there was little of which to be proud.

"During this week we have not heard from the Bobaths, but we all know of their work. The Bobaths are my friends, and they speak to you of neurology. It must be clear to all of you that they have something of value for the children of the world. For God's sake let us *use* it and bury forever the quarrels of the past.

"Let us get on with the job.

"It seems more than likely to me that my own job in South America is now drawing to a close.

"It is obvious that what bitter quarrels you once had, the volume of which prevented you from listening to each other, will now be replaced with honest minor disagreement and laudable discussion.

"I salute you as professional men and women of good will and I now leave you to your own highly capable leaders in South America, Drs. Veras, Brandão, Leitão, Fontes-Lima, Silva, Sequeiros, Brandt, Crespo, Porto and the rest.

"I shall look to you now to teach us in the future as we have been privileged to teach you in the past. I believe that the brilliant work of Drs. Raymundo and José Carlos Veras in the treatment of mongolism is simply the first in a long line of breakthroughs where the students will become the teachers.

"As for us, we must now turn our eyes to our own North America where the battles, quarrels and recriminations have raged longest and most intensely and to Europe where they are just beginning. We must work and hope and indeed pray that those of us responsible for the brain-injured child will find ourselves so busily engaged in finding new or better answers for these kids that there will remain ample time for discussion but no time at all for destructive and demeaning attacks on each other.

"It seems time now to put aside the endless theoretical discussions we have sometimes enjoyed and sometimes hated in the past three decades and examine some clear hard facts for, as interesting as theories are and as important as they may sometimes be, the fact remains that a theory which produces no result is worthless. Conversely, it is equally true that if a system produces real results, it may be reasonably argued that a theory to support it might not even be necessary.

"For a long time a great many of you have talked to me and written to me to tell me of your complete dissatisfaction with what has been happening to brain-injured children as a product of classical treatment and have asked me to tell you precisely what had been happening to the children we have been treating in Philadelphia using our program of neurological organization.

"It is a fair question which cries out for answering, but all of you who are involved in treatment and in statistical procedures appreciate just how difficult it is to answer that question.

"Ideally, such a report of results should be that arising from a rigorously controlled study, and the people of The Institutes have been unremitting in their efforts to obtain such a study. Many of you are personally aware of a good many of these efforts.

"At the present time such a study has been designed and planned in complete co-operation with Teaching Research which is a division of the Oregon State System of Higher Education. That carefully controlled study has been presented to the National Institutes of Health of the United States for approval and funding, and that application is presently under discussion with that agency. The results of that study will be presented as quickly as they are available.

"However, this study will require many years of time and the final results of that study will not be available until 1980 at the earliest.

"Neither parents nor those physicians and other professional people faced with the present reality of brain-injured children can wait for years to find the scientifically immaculate results of such studies.

"Indeed, even the organizations that saw fit to publish in 1968 a statement casting doubt on the work of The Institutes said in that statement, 'Advice to parents and professional workers cannot wait conclusive results of controlled studies of all aspects of the method.'

"My own Institutes in Philadelphia heartily concur with that statement, and we feel that it is incumbent upon us to make known precisely what is happening to children under treatment. We, of course, feel that it is incumbent upon all other groups treating brain-injured children by classical methods or any other method to do the same thing.

"It seems obvious that until controlled studies can be done, it is necessary that the advocates of all treatment methods, whether classical or not, make available some careful factual reports of what is actually happening to the children under treatment by that particular method. By so doing, it will be possible for parents and professionals alike to draw their own conclusions about significance and results of various methods until more scientific evidence is available."

I then went on to present the findings from two studies we had made, as follows:

"One study dealt with easily measurable physical factors. As previously mentioned, some remarkable physical changes are taking place in the severely brain-injured children being treated in The Philadelphia Institutes. As already pointed out, a very high percentage of brain-injured children are extremely small in physical size when compared to their chronological peers, but begin to grow at remarkably fast rates of speed when treatment is commenced.

"These observations of startling growth were first reported by Roselise Wilkinson, M.D., and Evan Thomas, M.D., both of The Institutes' staff, at a meeting of the American Academy of General Practice, Ohio Chapter, in August 1970.

"The particular study which I wish to summarize was done by Edward LeWinn, M.D., the medical director of the Research Institute of The Institutes for the Achievement of Human Potential in Philadelphia.

"In a study of 278 consecutively accepted brain-injured children under treatment at The Institutes in Philadelphia, he found that at onset of treatment 81.9 per cent of the children had chests smaller than the 50th percentile (i.e., were below average for their age), and 54.7 per cent of the children had chests below the 10th percentile (smallest 10 per cent of children).

"At the end of the study (after fourteen months of treatment) only 64.4 per cent of the children were now below average, and only 24.8 per cent remained in the lowest tenth. During the fourteen months of treatment their chests had grown at a rate which averaged 286 per cent of normal, and growth was continuing.

"In the course of treatment, 243 of the 278 children moved to a rate of chest growth that was above normal for their age, as follows:

Number growing	at less than 100% of normal					35
"	"	from 100% to 199% of normal				58
"	"	"	200% to 299% of normal			69
"	"	"	300% to 399% of normal			67
"	"	"	400% to 499% of normal			34
"	"	"	500% and over			15

"The story was much the same in terms of head growth. At the start of treatment 82.2 per cent of the 278 children had a head circumference below the 50th percentile. At the end of the study (fourteen months later) only 70.1 per cent were below average for their age.

"The average rate of growth in head circumference during the fourteen months of the study was 254 per cent of normal. At the end of the study the children were still under treatment and still continuing to grow in head size.

"In the course of treatment, 241 of the 278 children moved to a rate of growth in head circumference that was above normal for their age, as follows:

Number growing	at less than 100% of normal			37
"	"	" a rate between 100% and 199%		81
"	"	" a rate between 200% and 299%		82
"	"	" a rate between 300% and 399%		38
"	"	" a rate between 400% and 499%		18
"	"	" a rate of 500% and over		22

"Since these children ranged in age from 75 months to 198 months at the onset of treatment, and since each child was being compared in growth to his own exact chronological peers, it would appear that this remarkable change in growth rate had to be a product of the program of neurological organization.

"If these figures were being studied by workers in some field other than the human sciences, as for example by leaders in the Space Program, which is more pragmatic and more result-oriented than is our own, I believe that these results might be considered as constituting in themselves reasonable evidence that the program of neurological organization is substantially and favorably altering severely brain-injured children. As Thoreau has observed, 'Some circumstantial evidence is very strong, as when you find a trout in the milk.'

"I should now like to present another group of case histories, as follows:

"Two hundred and ninety brain-injured children applied for and were accepted for treatment during the year 1968 at The Institutes for the Achievement of Human Potential in Philadelphia, Pennsylvania. The children were actually treated daily at home by their parents. Parents and child returned no more often than every two months (and frequently less often) for re-evaluation of the child and revision of his program.

"Eliminated from the 290 children were ninety-five children who were under treatment for less than a year, since such children would have had, at the most, five visits and, at the least, no revisits at all; the staff is persuaded that five or less visits are seldom enough to give The Institutes' method a truly fair trial. It is, however, interesting that in those children eliminated, two had been discharged as functioning normally, while only one had been discharged as a failure. Also eliminated were twenty-five children under three years of age to remove the possibility that these children were simply "slow starters" who might yet have walked and talked without treatment.

"There were 170 children who met both the requirements of a year or more of programming and the age limit. They ranged from mildly brain-injured children who walked and talked, but badly, to profoundly brain-injured children who were unable to move or make sounds. Some of these were functionally completely blind or deaf. They ranged in age from thirty-six months to seventeen and one half years. The median age was 104 months. The mean age was 105.4 months.

AGE DISTRIBUTION CHART

Age	Number of Children
3 years	13
4 years	18
5 years	16
6 years	14
7 years	11
8 years	21
9 years	13
10 years	19
11 years	10
12 years	12
13 years	9
14 years	5
15 years	4
16 years or over	5

"Let me show you now the results we achieved with just one of these 170 children in terms of the following facts:

"First: *Initial Chronological Age.* This is simply the child's age in months, when we first saw him. In my example this was forty-three months.

"Second: *Initial Neurological Age.* This is determined through use of the Doman-Delacato Developmental Profile. In my example this was fifteen months.

"Third: *Initial Rate of Progress.* This is the ratio of initial neurological age to initial chronological age. In my example it is 15/43 or 36 per cent.

"Fourth: *Present Chronological Age.* In my example this is seventy-one months. In other words, he remained on program for twenty-eight months since he first came to us at age forty-three months.

"Fifth: *Present Neurological Age.* In my example this is thirty-four months. In other words, he gained nineteen months in neurological age since he came to us with an initial neurological age of fifteen months.

"Sixth: *Present Rate of Progress.* In my example this is 67.5 per cent, a figure derived from the ratio of his gain in neurological age while on program (nineteen months) to his gain in chronological age (twenty-eight months) while on program.

"Seventh: *Comparison of New Growth Rate with Old Growth Rate.* In my example this is 190 per cent, a figure derived from the ratio of his new growth rate (67.5) to his former growth rate (36).

"Eighth: *Estimated Time to Neurological Maturity at Normal Rate of Growth.* This is arrived at by taking this child's present neurological age (thirty-four months) and subtracting it from the seventy-two months that is assumed in the Profile to represent neurological maturity.

"Ninth: *Estimated Time to Neurological Maturity for this Child.* In my example this is given as fifty-six months—based on dividing the thirty-eight months that would be required at normal rate of growth by the child's present rate of progress (67.5 per cent of normal). In other words, *if he continues to progress at 67.5 per cent of normal*—he will net thirty-eight months of progress over the next fifty-six months of chronological time.

"We have on file the detailed results for the 170 children, [which we considered too much data for the average reader of this book]. Each example is summed up in a Comment. In my example we rate the outlook as Good inasmuch as this six-year-old, if he continues his present rate of progress, may well reach full neurological maturity by the time he is eleven years old. By contrast, we rate the next case in our file as Poor inasmuch as it would take that particular six-year-old nearly sixteen years to reach neurological maturity at his present rate.

"Other cases, depending on the indicated outlook, are rated Superb, Splendid, Excellent, Good, Fair, Poor or Impossible. These ratings don't necessarily reflect how well or poorly The Institutes' program has done for the child, but rather the probable chance of success, *assuming* continuing progress at the rate established during a year or more on the program.

"It must be stressed that the goal is seventy-two months of neurological age, i.e., competence to see, hear, feel, walk, talk, and do manual tasks as well as a fully normal six-year-old. When an individual reaches that level he may still be behind his peer group in terms of education and experience, but he will now be able to push ahead on these fronts as well as any normal individual—and will be able to catch up if we give him education and experience at an accelerated rate. We have found over and over again that a child with a really good tutor can learn as much in an hour as the average child learns in a day at school; as much in a day as the average child learns in a week at school.

"Overall, these 170 children had been on the program at the time of the study for a minimum of twelve months and a maximum of thirty-five months. The average time on program was twenty-four months. The outlook at the time of this study (i.e., after one to three years on program) was as shown in Fig. 24.

NUMBER OF CHIL- DREN	PER- CENTAGE OF ENTIRE GROUP	TIME REQUIRED FOR CHILD TO REACH NEUROLOGICAL MATURITY ASSUMING THE CONTINUATION OF PRESENT RATE OF GROWTH	OUTLOOK
61	35.9%	One month to 23 months	SUPERB
22	12.9%	24 months to 35 months	SPLENDID
13	7.6%	36 months to 47 months	EXCELLENT
5	2.9%	48 months to 59 months	GOOD
24	14.1%	60 months to 119 months	FAIR
17	10.5%	120 months to 191 months	POOR
28	16.5%	192 months and upward	PRESENTLY IMPOSSIBLE
—	—		
170			

FIGURE 24

"Among these 170 children, 146 highly important gains were made during the period of treatment. These gains were highly important by anyone's standards, even our own. These gains were:

5   children who could not walk were now walking.
17   children who could not talk were now talking.
3   children who were blind could now see.
    (Two of them could read, and I mean with their eyes.)
60   children who could not read could now read.
2   children who could not pick up objects with their hands could now do so.
35   children who could not write could now do so.
5   children who were deaf could now hear.
4   children who had seizures or convulsions no longer had them.

"Are such results good or bad?

"It depends, I believe, on whose standards you are using at which moment in history.

"This determination of how long it will take a child to reach normality is a critically important factor, because how long the parents can maintain their strength and determination is strongly related to how quickly a child is winning and how much longer treatment will take.

"It must be remembered that this determination is based on the *assumption* that this child will continue to grow at this rate. What we have done can be charted (Fig. 25), comparing him to normal.

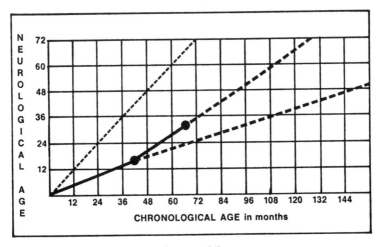

FIGURE 25

"The dotted line represents the average well child in his progress to neurological normality within the normal chronological time span.

"The solid line to the first dot at forty-three months of chronological age (and fifteen months of neurological age) represents the brain-injured child's growth (in my example) to the time we first saw him.

"The solid line to the second dot at seventy-one months of chronological age (and thirty-four months of neurological age) represents what has happened in the twenty-eight months he has been on program. By projecting the new line we can see that he will reach normalcy in about four and one half more years, *assuming* he continues this rate of growth.

"However, children seldom, if ever, grow at even rates of speed, which seems to invalidate such measurements as a means of making judgments. However, we actually see the child every two months and replot the child each visit so that we know precisely where we are. Sometimes the rate of growth increases. Sometimes it slows.

"In life a child's chart often looks like Figure 26, each of the dots representing a visit:

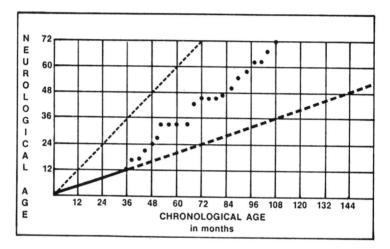

FIGURE 26

"Now we know:

1. Where the child was at the initial visit (prior to treatment).

2. How long it took him to get there.

3. His rate of progress prior to treatment.

4. Precisely where he is now, compared to himself prior to treatment.

5. How long it took him to get there.

6. His present rate of speed compared to his previous rate of speed.

7. His present rate of speed compared to an average well child.

8. How far he has yet to go to be functioning normally.

9. How long it will take him to get there with revaluations of that position every two months.

"That is a great deal to know as compared to the classical methods of measurement which generally tell us either nothing or, worse, something that isn't true. At best, they boil down to the less than scientific question, 'How do you think he looks today?' "

31.

WHERE DO WE GO FROM HERE?

It has been said that the only two difficult things about writing a book are to write the first sentence and to write the last sentence, and I have found it to be so.

I suppose the truth is that the last sentence is never really the final thing to be said, and I have left much unsaid. Some of what I have left unsaid remains unsaid because you have to stop somewhere if a book is ever to be done since clinical research is an ongoing thing and new discoveries happen every day. For that reason we have talked not at all about our most recent discoveries which are still being developed—and you have to stop somewhere.

There are also things of great importance which we understand and use but do not yet understand well enough to be able to explain them in all their complexities in a book. Included among these things are the full oxygen availability program, the spatial relations program, and others.

Still, we have covered much, and the parents of the brain-injured child who wish to begin him on a program certainly have enough important information to make a substantial difference in their child if they wish to do so—and that, I think, is a good thing.

Now I must ask myself where we are now. What of the past, what of the present and what of the future?

When the most senior members of our group began our work together more than thirty years ago we had never seen or heard of a single brain-injured child who had ever gotten well.

Things are a lot better than that now and along the long, long road that has run from then to now many, many kids have gotten well—more even than I remember. Instead of comparing our work with everyone else's, I much prefer to simply compare our own results of today with our own results back in the old days when we were using what are called, with a good deal too much dignity, "Classical Methods" of treatment. I must say that comparing us with us there is no comparison—for in those days nobody ever got well or even significantly better, and today many get well and a substantial majority get significantly better, and between *no* results and substantial results there is simply no comparison.

So, I must ask myself, how do I feel about it all these many years later? How do we all feel about it? Well, I think that the staff and all the people of The Institutes feel substantially overworked and substantially underpaid—in money, that is, but it's equally clear that you couldn't get rid of them with wild horses. I don't know anyone with whom they'd trade jobs. The truth is that the staff feels just a little sorry for everybody else.

I personally alternate between exultation and despair depending on which way I'm looking. When I remember those old days when no child ever made it and when it was considered immoral even to hope and when I compare that with the children who make it today, I am in sheer exultation and to look at the children who make it is little short of glorious.

But I cannot for the life of me exult too long because ever intruding on my thoughts are the kids who fail, even today, and they are far too many and there remain a few who are actually not changed at all, and when I think of these kids and their parents, who are often marvelous people, my exultation dissolves and I am left with the bleakest of despair because for these children, it is much as it was in the darkest days of centuries past.

So is today superb, or is it tragic? It is both, and which it is for each single child is a product of our knowledge and of our ignorance. Seldom, indeed, is the failure a product of the parents, who by and large are magnificent and who vary from each other only in the incredible amounts of strength they can muster to do routinely the difficult-to-do, frequent the unbelievable, and to do more often than occasionally—the impossible. Whoever said the impossible takes a little longer must have been speaking of parents. Sometimes it takes a *lot* longer.

So it is today and new discoveries not only continue to happen but indeed they are happening faster than ever they did before and at a breakneck pace as compared to the way they had happened to us in the beginning, and these new discoveries are daily changing the way things are for brain-injured kids. Today's results are unquestionably better than even the results we have reported in this book because they report on kids who started the program six long years ago and we know about new worlds since then. Today's kid unquestionably has a better chance than did the kid of six years ago. I would be more than surprised if tomorrow's child does not do better—far better than the boy or girl who starts today. Were it not better, I should stand not surprised but in open-mouthed astonishment.

Through the years, since kids first began to go all the way, each year has been better. Each year the number of successes has increased and the number of failures has declined, and so I believe it will continue to be in the future. Treatment will, I believe, become simpler and perhaps not so terribly demanding as it is today. So demanding is the program today that I know of only one thing in all the world that is more difficult—that is to have a child whom you love who can't do what other kids do. That is more difficult, and parents feel that the *worst* day on The Institutes' program is better than the *best* day when they have no answer. Still I think that our continuing discoveries will make things not quite so impossible as they sometimes seem to be today.

Surely one day we shall see the end in brain injury either because we shall have learned to solve it always or we shall see the end because we shall learn a better thing—how to prevent it. That will be a splendid day for the kids and parents alike as it will be a great day for the staff of The Institutes for the Achievement of Human Potential. But will it then be the end of all the long years of work with children? I think not. It is impossible to watch day by day as profoundly brain-injured children struggle their way upward to wellness without coming over and over again to a most startling conclusion. Consider it.

I offer you Child A (the average child). He is eight years of age and he performs at an average level, which is to say, he performs exactly in the middle of the group of children his own age.

Now I offer you Child B (the brain-injured child). When he was born he was severely brain-injured and had millions—indeed billions, of dead brain cells. We have taught his parents and they have treated him for five long years and today he is eight years of age and performs exactly as Child A, the average child, *yet Child B still has suffered the death of billions of brain cells.*

This we have seen over and over again. How long can we look at that without asking, What in the devil is wrong with *Child A* (not Child B).

Surely if Child B with billions of brain cells dead and gone can perform and function in every way as well as the average unhurt child, then there must be something wrong with Child A.

For many years we have made this inescapable observation.

Now we present Child C (Child C has had a hemispherectomy). When Child C was born he appeared to be perfectly normal but some time subsequent to his birth he suffered a blood clot on one side of his brain. By three years of age he was completely paralyzed on the right side of his body, his behavior was wild indeed and he was having overwhelming *grande-mal* convulsions. His condition was rapidly worsening and it was clear that unless something was done he was not going to survive. Something was done. Our neurosurgeon had surgically removed the left half of his brain. It was not alone the cortex which was removed but half his brain; everything, in fact, except two ancient sections called the thalamus and the head and tail of the caudate nucleus. Now Child C was eight years old and Child C could do everything that *Child A* could do.

How long could the brain surgeon look at that without saying to himself, What in the devil is wrong with *Child A*? Why can Child A with a whole brain not perform better than Child C who has half his brain in his head and half his brain in a jar?

For many years the neurosurgeon had made the same observation.

Why indeed should two children, B and C, with demonstrably profoundly injured brains be able to perform as well as Child A with a relatively uninjured brain.

When one has observed this and pondered this for many years he is led inescapably to a simple and clear conclusion. *The average child is not functioning half as well as he ought to be*, and everybody who has thought about it knows it. How else explain that phenomenon known as the P.T.A.

Where else do we see lay people telling the professionals how to do it. Everyone knows that something is wrong but nobody knows what. One father says that the school needs a swimming pool. A mother believes that the school day is too long—or too short. And so it goes. Everyone agrees only that something is wrong.

All over the world we have had opportunity to talk to groups of mothers and over and over again I have had opportunity to ask this question. "Will every mother in the room who thinks her child is doing as well as he or she could be, please put up your hand." The world over, no hand has been raised. Perhaps, I have said to myself, these are bashful mothers and so I have reversed the question. "Will every mother in the room who feels her child is *not* doing as well as he or she could be, please put up your hand." All hands go up.

Is it possible that mothers the world over are right in believing that well children are not doing as well as they should be doing?

Is it possible that average kids could be a great deal more effective than they are?

Is it possible that we have somehow vastly underestimated our children?

Is there any evidence that children could accomplish a great deal more than they are accomplishing?

There is indeed, and what is more they are considerably happier kids.

In Australia there are a couple of Olympic swimmers who teach infant babies to swim. Dr. Fay had long ago observed that if you put a one-day-old baby on his belly in a few inches of water he will hold his breath when his face is in the water and breathe when he lifts his head. Why not? He has been swimming, as it were, for the previous nine months. Three years ago we had the opportunity to visit the Timmermans in Melbourne to watch.

It was a joyous and beautiful thing to watch as a dozen lovely pink-skinned, bikini clad mothers splashed in the pool with as many pink-and-cream, two- and three-month-old infants. I shall not soon forget the lovely sight they made together as they individually bobbed their babies up and down in the very warm water of the large pool. Soon each mother was dropping her baby into the water while the child, with obvious enjoyment would swim to the surface to be caught up in mother's arms. They swam with gusto.

We photographed one little three-year-old, who has earned a Red Cross Life Saving Badge, as she towed her mother the length of the pool with ease and pride.

Her two-year-old brother insisted over and over again that I throw him into the deep end of the pool from which he would clamber and demand again that I throw him in until I and not he was too tired to continue the game.

Australia lies surrounded by seas and her name implies they are Southern seas. Is there then some genetic code deeply written into Australian children, some aquatic imperative that perforce makes them swim? But these children were not aborigines five generations earlier; their parents had trod England's green and pleasant land, and are Holland-born. To one not initiated to the potential of children it would appear strange.

I remember my friend John Eaglebull of Army days. John was a Sioux and a Chief at that. He was a college graduate as befitted a Sioux Chief, and since his name began with an E and mine a D we slept beside each other through Infantry Officer Candidate School. I remember the day that Eaglebull with great pride, showed me a snapshot of his two-year-old son. Looking at it made me nervous. Here was this tiny two-year-old boy sitting unassisted and alone on the back of a full-grown horse, with reins in hand.

I complained to Eaglebull that it was a dangerous thing to do.

"What is dangerous," demanded Eaglebull, "about taking a snapshot?"

"Suppose," I said, "the horse had moved."

"It would have spoiled the snapshot," Eaglebull said.

"But nobody is holding your son. He could have fallen off and fractured his skull," I explained.

"For Pete's sake, that's his horse," said Eaglebull patiently as if he were explaining to a child. "I don't know anybody at home who can remember when he couldn't ride a horse any more than you know anyone who can remember when he couldn't walk."

That superb teller of Indian-Cavalry stories and historian of the post-Civil War days, James Warner Bellah, once described the Sioux as "Five thousand of the world's finest light cavalry." And why not? Like my friend John Eaglebull and his son, they were born on horses.

Is this superb horsemanship not some equestrian imperative written on every plains Indian in some immutable genetic code over the hundreds of thousands of years that such codes take? It would seem so, for surely the Indians were superb horsemen—until one remembers that until the coming of the Spaniards, less than five hundred years ago, no American Indian had ever seen a horse.

More than ten years ago a man told me of a man in Japan, Dr. Shinichi Suzuki, who was supposed to have taught hundreds of two-, three- and four-year-old children to have played the violin. I am a musical incompetent and have never been able to so much as carry a tune, but I have friends who are first-rate musicians—among them Carl Delacato and Edward LeWinn and Suzy Wong, to name a few. They tell me that the violin is among the most difficult of instruments to master. The man who told me about the Japanese children playing the violin did not believe the story and was sure it was not possible for any three-year-old child to play the violin. I believed the story instantly since all my findings of the previous twenty years had led me to the conclusion that any tiny child can learn to do anything at all that an adult can present to him in a reasonable way. I was also persuaded that tiny children learned the most involved things imaginable (such as language) without the slightest effort.

Everything I knew had led me to the conclusion that when it comes to taking in raw data without the slightest effort, no adult could hold a candle to any two-year-old. I had, in fact, written Doman's First Law of Human Dynamics which stated that "All adults are hopelessly mentally retarded compared to any two-year-old."

Everything about the story fitted my own knowledge and my own biases. Naturally, I believed it. The man who told me the story and who did not believe it became visibly upset when I, who had never heard it before except from him, did believe it.

It was ten years before Hazel and I got to Matsumoto, Japan, to meet that genial genius, Dr. Suzuki. Dr. Suzuki had been kind enough to arrange a concert for us, and I must say that in a lifetime which has been most fortunately graced with lovely sights, few could compare with the sight of fifty tiny Japanese girls and boys of three to six years playing a two-hour concert not of "Old MacDonald Had a Farm" but instead of Bach, Mozart, Beethoven and Liszt. There remains in my memory of that moving afternoon at Talent Education a little four-year-old girl whose training was so advanced that she played the entire concert. She was on the front row of the stage and she played with great poise, enthusiasm and beauty. In the midst of a lovely concerto she stopped and quietly stooped to place her violin on the floor, at which time her mother came forward and they left the auditorium together. In a few minutes and before the concerto had ended she returned quietly to the stage and resumed playing.

It is the only time in my life I recall seeing a virtuoso leave the concert stage to go to the bathroom with her mother because while she played the violin superbly, she did not yet take care of herself in the bathroom alone.

Even now as I write my eyes grow blurred as I remember that day and thrill to the beauty of those superb and superbly happy children who glory in their enjoyment of playing.

The Japanese, of course, are an ancient people and as everyone knows extremely clever with their hands and with their brains and one thinks that surely there is written in some ancient genetic code a musical imperative that gives Japanese children a special license to play Beethoven on the violin—until one remembers that it is only slightly over a hundred years ago that the first Japanese ever set ear to Beethoven or eye to a violin.

Dr. Suzuki has by now taught more than eight thousand little children to play the violin. Eight thousand especially gifted children? Yes. Gifted only with a mother who brought each child to have the opportunity.

I have already spoken of how that brilliant man, Dr. Raymundo Veras, in Brazil taught a one-year-old girl to begin reading in three languages so that by the time she was three she could read entire books in Portuguese, English and German. You will remember that she was what is called a mongoloid. He has taught dozens of so-called mongoloid children to read before they are four years old. Around The Institutes that awful term mongoloid has been replaced. We call them Veras kids.

Much has been said about genetics in relation to those kids we used to call mongoloids, but I never met anyone in the world who believed they had a genetic advantage. Neither do I.

I love to ski, but since I learned to do so as an adult I am quite naturally a poor skier. I try to make up for my lack of ability with first-rate equipment and first-rate instructors, but it avails me little. I stand on the top of a slope and pretend to be admiring the scenery while in truth I am getting up my nerve. I stand with my expensive cap and my expensive Head skis, and if the truth be known I am sore afraid until behind me some five- or six-year-old yells, "Out of the way, Mister," and down the slope he tears with his barrel staves and rubber bands shusshing and slaloming. He can't pronounce them but can he do them!

Is it genetic to Vermont children? Easy as duck soup but not genetic. When I was a boy only the rich skied and that in Switzerland. Vermont made magnificent maple sugar.

In 1971 my book, *How To Teach Your Baby To Read,* was published in the twelfth language, Japanese, and a new world opened to me.

In Japan I found whole groups of true geniuses when I was invited by E.D.A. (Early Development Association) and the Japanese *Reader's Digest* to lecture in that beautiful land.

E.D.A. itself is a superb organization doing what I have long dreamed of seeing. It is a product of the fertile brains of brilliant Dr. Masaaki Honda, a pediatrician, Mr. Toshiyuki Miyamoto, a splendid editor, Mr. Masaru Ibuka, a genius whose brain recognizes no horizons. Not content with being the founder of the Sony Corporation and the chairman of the board, he has written the most charming book I have ever read. It is called, *Too Late in Kindergarten,* and is a must for all parents-to-be or parents of tiny children. Finally, there is Mr. Akira Tago, a first rate educator.

Vividly in my mind's eye do I remember my first visit to E.D.A. in Tokyo where for the first time I met my colleague, Professor Isao Ishii with whom I had long corresponded. Appropriately enough my first sight of that astonishing man was a view of him surrounded by a semicircle of two-, three- and four-year-old Japanese children who sat with their eyes riveted on his face. Although we had long awaited this moment, neither he nor I acknowledged each other in the slightest way lest the spell between him and the little kids be broken.

In Japan there are two written languages; one is Kanji which comes from the Chinese and which contains thousands of written characters that represent words, phrases or even sentences. This is the language of the scholars and of literate adults. The other language is Kana and this is a simplified Japanese alphabet having forty-eight characters. It had always been assumed that grade school children could not learn Kanji but only Kana, though high school children learned Kanji.

Professor Ishii had begun as a university professor and had quite properly worked his way upward to being a kindergarten teacher. He had quite properly learned that children could learn Kanji quite as easily as they learned Kana and a good deal easier than adults. Having read my book he had experimented with teaching tiny children and older "mentally retarded" children Kanji. He was delighted to find that the smaller the children were, the easier it was to read Kanji.

Now at last I was face to face with him. At the level of his forehead he held a series of cards about ten inches square and on each of them was printed a Kanji character. All eyes watched intently. Suddenly he exposed a card for a split second. So briefly was it seen that I had no clear mental picture of this complex Chinese character. "Monkey" shouted the tiny children in unison. "Bird," "Automobile," "Hand," "Foot," "Mother," "Father," "Banana," and so it went through thirty or forty characters shown at random. Not only were these tiny children reading and reading easily and joyously, but they were reading the complex Kanji and not the simplified Kana.

In another room we watched the tiny children paint under the direction of a great Japanese illustrator. They painted joyfully and splendidly. They painted not with their fingers but with brushes, and they painted in oils.

In still another room we saw a semicircle of two-, three- and four-year-olds surrounding an attractive young American girl whose virtue was that she spoke no Japanese but only English. Hazel and I watched with rapture while she and the children carried on an elegant English conversation.

Here was in reality a dream we had long dreamed. Our hearts pounded and our spirits soared.

E.D.A. was doing much that we had so long known was possible.

Had not we long ago taught tiny children to read, even severely brain-injured ones? Had not we taught tiny children to do a fascinating instant mathematics that no staff member could match?

Did not I have a precious possession in the form of hundreds of letters from mothers the world over reporting to me what had happened to their little boys and girls after they had taught them to read?

Is it not true that when the world begins to bother me I go to my office and lock the door and read the letters my mothers have written me about their children, both well and brain-injured?

Do not those letters restore my soul in their unselfishness and their singleness of purpose in giving their children a better tomorrow.

Is it not obvious that Australian children have no corner on swimming nor Sioux children on horses, Vermont kids on skiing, Philadelphia kids on reading, Japanese children on violins, and so on and so on and so on the world over.

Is it not obvious that *all* children can be *all* things, and that giving them the opportunity to develop their brains is a joyous process for mother and child alike?

It's hard to imagine what the world will be like tomorrow when everyone knows the truth about little kids and every child has his or her opportunity to know all the magnificent things there are to know and is able to do all the great things there are to do.

What we have to do to bring about that lovely day—but there I go trying to say all there is to say in a single book and finding it impossible to write that last sentence. The problem is that this book is about how to make brain-injured children well. From doing that we've learned how to make well children weller—but that's really another story, isn't it?

APPENDIX A
MORE INFORMATION

COURSES:

What to Do About Your Brain-Injured Child
How to Multiply Your Baby's Intelligence

WHAT TO DO ABOUT YOUR BRAIN-INJURED CHILD CATALOG:

The Programs of the Institutes

HOW TO TEACH YOUR BABY CATALOG:

The Gentle Revolution Catalog

MATERIALS:

How to Teach Your Baby to Read Kit
How to Teach Your Baby Math Kit

THE GENTLE REVOLUTION SERIES VIDEOS:

How to Teach Your Baby to Read
How to Give Your Baby Encyclopedic Knowledge
How to Teach Your Baby Math

CHILDREN'S BOOKS:

The Life and Times of Inigo McKenzie Series
Nose is Not Toes

FOR MORE INFORMATION CALL OR WRITE:

The Registrar
The Institutes for the Achievement of Human Potential
8801 Stenton Avenue
Philadelphia, PA 19118 U.S.A.

1-800-344-MOTHER
1-215-233-2050

APPENDIX B

Reprinted from the *Journal of The American Medical Association,*
September 17, 1960, Vol. 174, pp. 257–62,
Copyright 1960, by American Medical Association.

A new system has been developed for the treatment of children with severe brain injuries. This concept, based on neurological organization, is aimed at the injured central nervous system rather than at the resultant peripheral symptoms. The authors devised a developmental mobility scale which described 13 levels of normal development as the criteria of progress during a two-year study of 76 children. The program consisted of permitting the child normal developmental opportunities in areas where the responsible brain level was undamaged, externally imposing the bodily patterns of activity which were the responsibility of damaged brain levels, establishment of hemispheric dominance and early unilaterality, respiratory improvement as measured by vital capacity, and sensory stimulation to improve bodily awareness and position sense. The results of this study are significantly better than those achieved by the authors with previous methods.

CHILDREN WITH SEVERE BRAIN INJURIES
Neurological Organization in Terms of Mobility

Robert J. Doman, M.D., Eugene B. Spitz, M.D., Philadelphia, Elizabeth Zucman, M.D., Paris, Carl H. Delacato, Ed.D., and Glenn Doman, P.T., Philadelphia

The large number of conferences, seminars, and publications regarding the brain-injured child indicates not so much the volume of new information available but rather the intensity of the search for new information.

We had long been dissatisfied with the results of our own methods of treatment and believed that the time requirements in treating children with severe brain injuries could scarcely be justified in light of the low percentage of marked successes as compared with children who were essentially without treatment.

During 1956 and 1957 we developed a new approach to such cases, the goal of which was to establish in brain-injured children the developmental stages observed in normal children. The program, which aimed at both normal and damaged brain levels, consisted of: (*a*) permitting the child normal developmental opportunities in areas in which the responsible brain level was undamaged; (*b*) externally imposing the bodily patterns of activity which were the responsibility of damaged brain levels; and (*c*) utilizing additional factors to enhance neurological organization.

The team used consisted of a physiatrist, a neurosurgeon, an orthopedic surgeon, a nurse, a physical therapist, and a psychologist. In 1958, a two-year outpatient study was begun which used these developmental stages in the treatment of 76 brain-injured children. Each patient was seen bimonthly.

MATERIAL

Subjects—This study of 76 children includes every child seen in the Children's Clinic during the study period who met the following criteria: 1. The existence of brain injury. (For the purpose of this study, brain-injured children are defined as those children whose lesion lies in the brain. The definition includes both traumatic and nontraumatic lesions but excludes children who are genetically defective.) 2. A minimum of six months' treatment. 3. No child was eliminated because of the severity of his involvement.

Diagnosis of Brain Pathology—The diagnosis was made after neurological examination and, in most patients, after an EEG (36), air study (42), and subdural tap (22) had been done. The group of 76 was composed of children who had spasms, athetosis, ataxia, rigidities, tremors, and mixed symptoms; 24 of these children had clinical seizures.

Classification of Brain Pathology—The brain pathology was classified as to type, location, and degree in the following manner.

1. Type: (*a*) unilateral brain damage: This group contained 15 children with either subdural hematoma (all operated on), vascular malformation, or hemiatrophy of nonspecific causation. Of these 15 children, 4 had hemispherectomies performed by us; (*b*) bilateral

brain damage: This group contained 61 children with conditions such as hydrocephalus, subdural hematoma (all operated on), kernicterus, postencephalitic damage, dysgenesis of corpus callosum, dysgenesis of cerebellum, dysgenesis of cortex, porencephaly, or diffuse cortical atrophy of nonspecific causation. We performed 14 ventriculojugular and 2 ventriculoperitoneal shunts on the 16 hydrocephalic patients. The therapeutic program was instituted no sooner than 10 months after surgery.

2. Location: Upon air study, 30 children demonstrated dilation of the lateral ventricles, and 12 demonstrated dilation of the entire ventricular system, thus indicating the presence of subcortical as well as cortical damage. Locating these lesions in terms of the Phelps-Fay classification,[1] there were 61 cerebral lesions (spastic patients), 12 midbrain lesions (athetoid patients), three basal ganglion lesions

TABLE 1.

Stage	Level	Mobility	No. of Children
Movement	0	None.	20
	1	Rolling over	17
	2	Circling or going backward	2
Crawling	3	Moving forward flat on abdomen without pattern.	5
	4	Homologously.	4
	5	Homolaterally.	3
	6	Cross pattern	2
Creeping	7	Without pattern	1
	8	Homologously.	2
	9	Homolaterally.	0
	10	Cross pattern	0
Walking	11	Pulling up to erect position holding on to furniture & standing, holding onto furniture	0
	12	Walking without help, without pattern	20
	13	Walking, cross pattern	0

FIGURE 27

(two patients with tremor, one with rigidity), and 10 cerebellar lesions (ataxic patients).

3. Degree: Both clinical examination and neurosurgical diagnostic procedures indicated that the degree of brain damage ranged from mild to severe. No child was eliminated from this study due to severity of either clinical symptoms or degree of brain pathology.

Age at Beginning of Study—The ages ranged from 12 months to nine years, with a median age of 26 months and a mean age of 30 months. The children were separated into three age groups of developmental significance: 0–18 months, 16 children; 18–36 months, 41 children; and over 36 months, 19 children.

Level and Stages of Movement at Beginning of Therapy—The level of movement was defined according to a modification of the developmental patterns of Gesell and co-workers[2-3] and Fay,[4-5] and these were numerically designated for reference purposes. The stages described are: (*a*) moving arms and legs without forward movements, (*b*) crawling, (*c*) creeping, and (*d*) walking (Table 1). In our experience, each stage described was dependent on the successful completion of the previous stage.

IQ, Affect, and Speech—No child was eliminated because of severity of deficiency in these areas.

Duration of Treatment—The duration of treatment ranged from 6 to 20 months, with a mean of 11 months.

METHOD

After thorough neurological studies, the children were evaluated to determine their disabilities in functional terms. An outpatient program of neurological organization was then prescribed and taught to the parents. The parents were required to carry out the program exactly as prescribed. The children's course was reviewed by the team on an average of every two months, and treatment changes were made to correspond to new developmental levels of accomplishment. The treatment consisted of two types.

Treatment Type I—All nonwalking children (56) were required to spend all day on the floor in the prone position and were encouraged to crawl (prone method) or creep (hand-knee method) when that level of accomplishment was possible. The only permissible exceptions were to feed, love, and treat the child. This increased the opportunity for the reproduction of the normal functional-positional situation of a healthy child during the first 13 months of life.

Treatment Type II—In each case, at that level of accomplishment at which pathology precluded the child's advancement to the next developmental stage, a specific pattern of activity was prescribed which passively imposed on the central nervous system the functional activity which was normally the responsibility of that damaged brain level. Initially these patterns were in some cases partially, and in other cases completely, those which had been described by Fay.[4] As time passed, our team discontinued some of these, modified others, and added those which it believed to be useful. Each of these patterns had its counterpart in the normal developmental growth of a healthy child so well described by Gesell and Amatruda.[2] The children were patterned for five minutes, four times daily, seven days a week without exception. The patterns were administered by three adults. One adult turned the head, another moved the right arm and leg, and the third moved the left arm and leg. The patterns were to be performed smoothly and rhythmically at all levels.

Activity Pattern I (Homolateral): Children who could not crawl

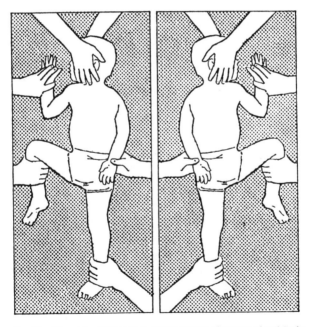

Fig. 28.—Homolateral Patterning: demonstration of pattern of activity in treatment of children with severe brain injuries who cannot crawl.

FIGURE 28

(44) and those who crawled below cross-pattern level (7) were patterned in the homolateral pattern, which was accomplished by one adult turning the head while the adult on the side to which the head was turned flexed the arm and leg. The adult on the opposite side extended both limbs. As the head was turned, the flexed limbs extended while the extended limbs flexed (Fig. 28).

Activity Pattern II (Cross Pattern): Children who could crawl in cross pattern or who could creep (5) were patterned in cross pattern, which was accomplished by one adult turning the head, while the adult on the side toward which the head was turned flexed the arm and extended the leg. The adult on the opposite side extended the arm and flexed the leg. When the head was turned, the position of the limbs was reversed (Fig. 29).

Activity Pattern III (Cross Pattern): Children who walked but poorly (20) were also patterned at the cross-pattern level.

Treatment for Neurological Organization—To enhance neurological

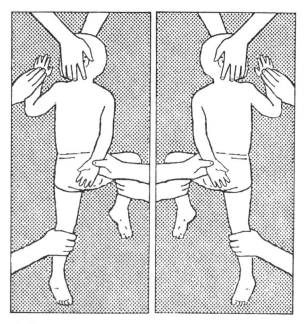

Fig. 29. — Cross-pattern Patterning: demonstration of activity in treatment of children who can crawl or creep, or walk but poorly.

FIGURE 29

organization, the children were evaluated in the light of the functions described below, and a treatment program was devised. The program included the following stages: 1. When tests showed sensory losses or when results of tests were indefinite due to communication problems, the children were placed on a program of sensory stimulation which included application of heat and cold, brushing, pinching, and establishment of body image appreciation by letting the child experience the relationship between his hand and his face, his hand and his mother's face, and similar relationships. 2. As each child reached the point where laterality influenced neurological organization, a program to establish dominance was instituted. 3. A breathing program to improve vital capacity was prescribed. All other therapy and use of mechanical aids were discontinued, except for anticonvulsant medication when indicated.

TABLE 2.

Level	Children at Beginning of Study		Children at End of Study	
	No.	%	No.	%
0	20	26.3	0	0.0
1	17	22.4	0	0.0
2	2	2.6	6	7.9
3	5	6.6	9	11.8
4	4	5.3	4	5.3
5	3	3.9	5	6.6
6	2	2.6	5	6.6
7	1	1.4	3	3.9
8	2	2.6	0	0.0
9	0	0.0	1	1.3
10	0	0.0	8	10.5
11	0	0.0	4	5.3
12	20	26.3	7	9.2
13	0	0.0	24	31.6
Total	76	100.0	76	100.0

FIGURE 30

RESULTS

The results were evaluated according to the following categories: (1) global results, (2) results in the light of chronological age, (3) results in the light of the individual disposition of each patient, and (4) results in the light of the functional level at the onset of the program.

Global Results—The mean improvement of mobility was 4.2 levels. The mean level of mobility was 4.4 at the beginning of the program and 8.6 at the end of the program. The range of improvement was 0 to 13 levels. If we consider perfect walking the potential for every child, the group achieved 51% of this goal (Table 2 and Fig. 30).

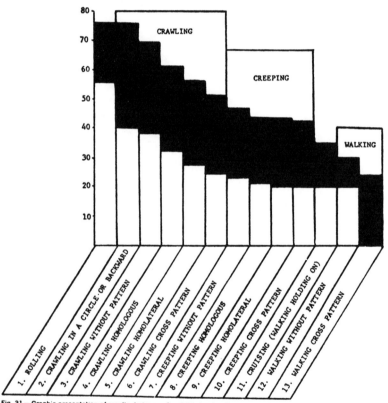

Fig. 31—Graphic presentation of results, in terms of mobility levels, of treatment of children with severe brain injuries.

FIGURE 31

The following findings are of interest: Of the 20 children unable to move and the 17 unable to walk, none remained at these stages. Twelve children were ready to walk at the end of the study. Eight were creeping cross pattern (level 10), and four were holding onto objects (level 11).

Eight of the group who could walk initially improved significantly in their walking but did not become perfect and, therefore, could not be considered as having increased their functional competence by one level. All but two of the other children improved by one or more levels.

Eleven children learned to walk completely independently. All but two of these had begun treatment at, or before, two years of age, and all achieved completely independent walking in less than 12 months of treatment. The functional level of this group at the beginning of the study was virtually the same as the level of the other 65 children. The entire group mean level at the outset was 4.4, compared with a mean of 4.1 for this group of 11 who learned to walk independently.

Only six children were discharged, all of whom had learned to walk perfectly; three of these had been walking poorly and three had been unable to walk at the beginning of the program. The other 8 who had learned to walk and the other 17 who had improved in walking were not discharged because of residual problems in speech or behavior.

Results in Light of Chronological Age—The children were separated into three age groups of developmental significance for purposes of evaluation. There was no significant difference of mean improvement among the three different age groups (Table 3).

Individual Results in Light of Functional Level at Beginning of Study—An analysis of the original level-ultimate level disposition of each case indicates an over-all improvement of 4.1 levels within the study. The improvement in individual patients is shown in Table 4.

Rate of Improvement in Light of Functional Level at Beginning of Study—The levels of improvement were evaluated by analysis of 13 levels in terms of functional components (Table 5).

COMMENT

We found significant improvement when we compared the results of the classic procedures we had previously followed with the results of the procedures described above. It is our opinion that the signifi-

TABLE 3.*

No.	Age, Mo.	Improvement		
		In Stages, Mean	Maximum Possible	% of Potential Achieved
16	Under 18	5.0	10.8	46
41	18 to 36	4.1	8.2	50
19	Over 36	3.2	6.7	47

* Numerical representations correspond to 13 stages of development described above.

FIGURE 32

cance of the difference tends to corroborate the validity of the hypothesis set up as the theoretical basis of the program.

These procedures are based on the premise that certain brain levels, i.e., pons, midbrain and cortex, have separate, consecutive responsibilities in terms of mobility. The goal of these procedures (neurological organization) is to create a climate in which a brain-injured child may develop and utilize those brain levels which are uninjured as they are developed in the normal child concurrent with myelinization during the first 18 months of life.[6]

We have observed that the opportunities to crawl and creep are rarely accorded to the brain-injured child. Great emphasis should be placed on permitting the brain-injured child to remain on the floor, which Gesell and co-workers have described as the normal child's "athletic field," thus giving the child an opportunity to utilize and exploit uninjured brain levels and achieve the functions for which such brain levels are responsible.

After neurological examination and testing had established the level of brain injury, we imposed on the child's central nervous system patterns of activity which have as their goal the reproduction of normal activities which would have been the product of the injured brain level had it not been injured. The pattern aspect of the procedure was achieved after a study and modification of Fay's work with the brain-injured child and Gesell's work with the normal child and was then integrated into the procedure developed by us.

It is our opinion that to be successful in such a program, the procedure must be carried out "wholistically." While we placed varying

TABLE 4.

No.	No. of Children in Each at Beginning	Level at End of Study													
		0	1	2	3	4	5	6	7	8	9	10	11	12	13
0	20	..	..	5	4	3	2	..	1	..	1	1	..	1	2
1	17	..	..	2	1	1	2	4	1	..	..	4	2	..	..
2	2	..	..	..	1	. .	..	..	..	..	..	1	..	..	..
3	5	..	..	..	2	..	1	1	..	..	..	1	..	..	..
4	4	..	..	..	..	..	..	..	..	..	..	..	2	2	..
5	3	..	..	..	..	..	..	..	1	..	..	..	..	1	1
6	2	..	..	..	..	..	..	..	..	..	..	..	..	2	..
7	1	..	..	..	..	..	..	..	..	..	..	1	..	..	..
8	2	..	..	..	..	..	..	..	..	..	..	..	..	..	2
9		..	..	..	..	..	..	..	..	..	..	..	..	..	..
10		..	..	..	..	..	..	..	..	..	..	..	..	..	..
11		..	..	..	..	..	..	..	..	..	..	..	..	..	..
12	20	..	..	..	..	..	..	..	..	..	..	..	..	8	12
13		..	..	..	..	..	..	..	..	..	..	..	..	..	..
Totals	76	..	..	7	8	6	5	5	3	..	1	8	4	14	17

FIGURE 33

emphasis upon the importance of different areas within the program, it was our experience that success could not be achieved by using the components of the program in isolation.

We believe that the program must include: (a) the opportunity for the brain-injured child to spend prolonged periods on the floor in the prone or quadruped position, so that he may crawl or creep in order to utilize uninjured brain areas in physiological development. Given this opportunity, the brain-injured child may advance several developmental levels unaided; (b) the utilization of patterns of activity administered passively to a child which reproduce the mobility functions for which injured brain levels are responsible; (c) a program of sensory stimulation to make the child body-conscious in terms of position sense and proprioception. We believe that sensory reception

TABLE 5.*

Functional Level	Improvement		
	In Levels, Mean	Maximum Possible	% of Potential Achievement
No mobility	5.8	13.0	43
Rolling	5.7	12.0	47
Circling	4.5	11.0	45
Moving straight without pattern . . .	2.4	10.0	24
Crawling	6.5	8.0	80
Creeping	4.3	5.3	80
Walking	0.8	1.0	80

* Numerical representations correspond to 13 levels of development described above.

FIGURE 34

is a prerequisite to motor expression; (*d*) a program of establishing cortical hemispheric dominance through the development of unilateral handedness, footedness and "eyedness." This was instituted when a lack of neurological organization at this level so indicated;[7] and (*e*) the institution of a breathing program to achieve the maximal vital capacity, since, in our experience, we had observed the restricted vital capacity and the recurrence of respiratory difficulties in many brain-injured children.

While we think that this program resulted in benefits to the children studied in the areas of language and affect, we confined this report to results achieved in terms of mobility. A later report will deal with the results achieved in other areas by this program of neurological organization.

We wish to stress the fact that no child was eliminated from the study due to initial lack of affect or mobility. It can be observed from the facts presented that many of the children, when initially evaluated, showed little affect and no mobility, and that a large number of them made significant progress. It should also be stressed that during the study all other programs of therapy or habilitation were discontinued and that no mechanical aids, such as braces or crutches, were used.

We place emphasis upon the fact that the children studied were evaluated and treated with reference to the central neurological lesion rather than upon the symptomatic results of the central lesion.

It is our opinion that the results of this study, when compared with the results of our previous work, are sufficiently encouraging to warrant an expanded and continued study of these procedures.

We do not believe that all the techniques which would be useful in achieving neurological organization have been developed by this study. We think that many additional techniques may be developed which could speed the process of habilitation of children with severe brain injuries and perhaps increase the number of types of brain injuries which can be treated. Later reports will deal with the results of studies being conducted at the time of writing.

SUMMARY

A two-year study was conducted on 76 brain-injured children. Its goal was to determine whether a program aimed at neurological organization would be productive of greater results in terms of mobility than we had previously achieved by more classic therapy.

The children studied were both evaluated and treated in light of their central neurological lesions in a program which we had devised to utilize undamaged brain levels to achieve the physiological functions for which such levels are responsible and to assist children at damaged brain levels in achieving function, as far as possible, by means of a program designed to reproduce normal activity. The preliminary results of this study are encouraging. Further studies of these procedures will be undertaken.

8801 Stenton Ave. (18) (Dr. R. J. Doman).

Thanks are due to Lieut. Col. Anthony R. Flores (MSC), Rosemary Warnock, R.N., and Lindley C. Boyer, staff members of the Children's Clinic, whose work and technical assistance made this study possible. Mr. Lloyd P. Wells, staff photographer, made all photographs necessary to this study.

REFERENCES

1. Abbott, M. *Syllabus of Cerebral Palsy Treatment Techniques.* New York: College of Physicians and Surgeons, Columbia University, May 1953, p. 10.

2. Gesell, A. L., and Amatruda, C. S. *Developmental Diagnosis: Normal and Abnormal Child Development,* Ed. 2. New York: Harper & Brothers, 1947, Chap. 11.

3. Gesell, A. L., and others. *Infant and Child in Culture of Today: Guidance of Development in Home and Nursery School.* New York: Harper & Brothers, 1943.

4. Fay, T. "Neurophysical Aspects of Therapy in Cerebral Palsy," *Archives of Physical Medicine.* 29:327–34 (June) 1948.

5. Fay, T. "Origin of Human Movement," *American Journal of Psychiatry,* III: 644–52 (March) 1955.

6. Thomas, A., and Dargassies, S. A. *Etudes neurologiques sur le nouveau-né et le jeune nourrisson.* Paris: Masson, 1952.

7. Delacato, C. H. *Treatment and Prevention of Reading Problems: (Neuro-Psychological Approach).* Springfield, Ill.: Charles C. Thomas, Publisher, 1959.

INDEX

OTHER RELATED BOOKS, VIDEOS & KITS IN THE GENTLE REVOLUTION SERIES

Glenn Doman has demonstrated, time and time again, that very young children are far more capable of learning than we ever imagined. He has taken his remarkable work—work that explores why children from birth to age six learn better and faster than older children do—and given it practical application. As the founder of The Institutes for the Achievement of Human Potential, he has created home programs that any parent can follow.

HOW TO TEACH YOUR BABY TO READ
Glenn Doman and Janet Doman

How to Teach Your Baby to Read provides your child with the skills basic to academic success. It shows you just how easy and pleasurable it is to teach a young child to read. It explains how to begin and expand the reading program, how to make and organize your materials, and how to more fully develop your child's potential. *Paperback $9.95 / Hardback $18.95*

Also available: **How To Teach Your Baby To Read™ Video Tape**
How To Teach Your Baby To Read Kit

HOW TO TEACH YOUR BABY MATH

Glenn Doman and Janet Doman

How to Teach Your Baby Math instructs you in successfully developing your child's ability to think and reason. It shows you just how easy and pleasurable it is to teach a young child math. It explains how to begin and expand the math program, how to make and organize your materials, and how to more fully develop your child's potential. *Paperback $9.95 / Hardback $15.95*

Also available: **How To Teach Your Baby Math™ Video Tape**
How To Teach Your Baby Math Kit

HOW TO GIVE YOUR BABY ENCYCLOPEDIC KNOWLEDGE

Glenn Doman

How to Give Your Baby Encyclopedic Knowledge provides a program of visually stimulating information designed to help your child take advantage of his or her natural potential to learn anything. It shows you just how easy and pleasurable it is to teach a young child about the arts, science, and nature. Your child will recognize the insects in the garden, know the countries of the world, discover the beauty of a painting by Van Gogh, and more. It explains how to begin and expand your program, how to make and organize your materials, and how to more fully develop your child's mind. *Paperback $9.95 / Hardback $19.95*

Also available: **How To Give Your Baby Encyclopedic Knowledge™ Video Tape**
How To Give Your Baby Encyclopedic Knowledge Kit

HOW TO MULTIPLY YOUR BABY'S INTELLIGENCE
Glenn Doman and Janet Doman

How to Multiply Your Baby's Intelligence provides a comprehensive program that will enable your child to read, to do mathematics, and to learn about anything and everything. It shows you just how easy and pleasurable it is to teach your young child, and to help your child become more capable and confident. It explains how to begin and expand this remarkable program, how to make and organize your materials, and how to more fully develop your child's potential. *Paperback $12.95 / Hardback $24.95*

Also available: **How To Multipy Your Baby Intelligence™ Kit**

HOW TO TEACH YOUR BABY TO BE PHYSICALLY SUPERB
Glenn Doman, Douglas Doman and Bruce Hagy

How to Teach Your Baby to Be Physically Superb explains the basic principles, philosophy, and stages of mobility in easy-to-understand language. This inspiring book describes just how easy and pleasurable it is to teach a young child to be physically superb. It clearly shows you how to create an environment for each stage of mobility that will help your baby advance and develop more easily. It shows that the team of mother, father, and baby is the most important athletic team your child will ever be a part of. It explains how to begin, how to make your materials, and how to expand your program. This complete guide also includes full-color charts, photographs, illustrations, and detailed instructions to help you create your own program. *Hardback $24.95*

WHAT TO DO ABOUT
YOUR BRAIN-INJURED CHILD

Glenn Doman

In this breakthrough book, Glenn Doman—pioneer in the treatment of the brain-injured—brings real hope to thousands of children, many of whom are inoperable, and many of whom have been given up for lost and sentenced to a life of institutional confinement. Based upon the decades of successful work performed at The Institutes for the Achievement of Human Potential, the book explains why old theories and techniques fail, and why The Institutes philosophy and revolutionary treatment succeed. *Paperback $11.95 / Hardback $19.95*

CHILDREN'S BOOKS

About the Books

Very young readers have special needs. These are not met by conventional children's literature which is designed to be read by adults *to* little children not *by* them. The careful choice of vocabulary, sentence structure, printed size, and formatting is needed by very young readers. The design of these children's books is based upon more than a quarter of a century of search and discovery of what works best for very young readers.

ENOUGH, INIGO, ENOUGH

written by Janet Doman   illustrated by Michael Armentrout

Young upstart Inigo McKenzie tells us in his own words about his early life. Familiar voculary and bold 1/2 inch print make this little book a breeze for children 1 to 6. *Hardcover $14.95*

NOSES IS NOT TOES
written by Glenn Doman   illustrated by Janet Doman

This clever little reader combines charming and familiar rhyme words with a story about all sorts of interesting creatures. Ages 1 to 3. *Hardcover $14.95*

THE MOOSE BOOK
written by Janet Doman   illustrated by Michael Armentrout

The story of a young moose's successful struggle to overcome illiteracy with the help of his mother and a cast of other friends. Ages 2 to 6. *Paperback $9.95*

THE WRONG COCKATIEL
written by Michael Armentrout

The somewhat embroidered tale of a young woman who buys a cockatiel as a pet and is given the wrong one. Ages 3 to 6. *Paperback $9.95*

NANKI GOES TO NOVA SCOTIA
written by Michael Armentrout

The almost true story of a young dog's visit to a foreign land, and his adventures along the way. For ages 3 to 6. Paperback $9.95

For a complete catalog of Avery books, call us at 1-800-548-5757.

COURSE OFFERINGS AT THE INSTITUTES

HOW TO MULTIPY YOUR BABY'S INTELLIGENCE™ COURSE

The Institutes offer a one week certification course for parents, expectant parents, and grandparents. This course encompasses reading, mathematics, encyclopedic knowledge, physical development, nutrition, and the instruction of foreign language and music.

WHAT TO DO ABOUT YOUR BRAIN-INJURED CHILD COURSE

The Institutes offer a five-day course exclusively for the parents of brain-injured children or the relatives of brain-injured adults. This course teaches parents the basic principles of brain growth and development. It enables parents to learn how to evaluate their children and design a home program to help their children develop intellectually, physically, phsiologically and socially. For more information call or write:

The Institutes for the Achievement of Human Potential
8801 Stenton Avenue
Philadelphia, PA 19118 USA

1-800-344-MOTHER or 1-215-233-2050
or FAX 1-215-233-3940